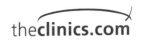

PSYCHIATRIC CLINICS
OF NORTH AMERICA

Clinical Interviewing: Practical Tips from Master Clinicians

GUEST EDITOR
Shawn Christopher Shea, MD

June 2007 • Volume 30 • Number 2

SAUNDERS

An Imprint of Elsevier, Inc.
PHILADELPHIA   LONDON   TORONTO   MONTREAL   SYDNEY   TOKYO

W.B. SAUNDERS COMPANY
A Division of Elsevier Inc.

1600 John F. Kennedy Boulevard · Suite 1800 · Philadelphia, PA 19103-2899

http://www.theclinics.com

PSYCHIATRIC CLINICS OF NORTH AMERICA   Volume 30, Number 2
June 2007   ISSN 0193-953X
Editor: Sarah E. Barth   ISBN-13: 978-1-4160-4362-1
                                                             ISBN-10: 1-4160-4362-4

Psychiatric Clinics of North America (ISSN 0193-953X) is published quarterly by Elsevier Inc., 360 Park Avenue South, New York, NY 10010-1710. Months of issue are March, June, September, and December. Business and Editorial Offices: 1600 John F. Kennedy Blvd., Suite 1800, Philadelphia, PA 19103-2899. Customer Service Office: 6277 Sea Harbor Drive, Orlando, FL 32887-4800 Periodicals postage paid at New York, NY and additional mailing offices. Subscription prices are $194.00 per year (US individuals), $329.00 per year (US institutions), $97.00 per year (US students/residents), $232.00 per year (Canadian individuals), $400.00 per year (Canadian Institutions), $270.00 per year (foreign individuals), $400.00 per year (foreign institutions), and $135.00 per year (international & Canadian students/residents). Foreign air speed delivery is included in all *Clinics'* subscription prices. All prices are subject to change without notice. **POSTMASTER:** Send address changes to *Psychiatric Clinics of North America,* Elsevier Periodicals Customer Service, 6277 Sea Harbor Drive, Orlando, FL 32887-4800. Customer Service: 1-800-654-2452 (US). From outside of the US, call 1-407-345-4000.

Psychiatric Clinics of North America is covered in *Index Medicus, Current Contents/Social and Behavioral Sciences, Social Science Citation Index, Embase/Excerpta Medica,* and PsycINFO.

Printed in the United States of America.

Clinical Interviewing: Practical Tips from Master Clinicians

GUEST EDITOR

SHAWN CHRISTOPHER SHEA, MD, Director, Training Institute for Suicide Assessment and Clinical Interviewing, Stoddard; and Adjunct Assistant Professor of Psychiatry, Dartmouth Medical School, Hanover, New Hampshire

CONTRIBUTORS

BRUCE BAKER, EdD, Training Institute for Suicide Assessment, Stoddard, New Hampshire

CHRISTINE BARNEY, MD, Adjunct Assistant Professor of Psychiatry, Dartmouth Medical School, Hanover, New Hampshire

JAMES BOEHNLEIN, MD, Professor of Psychiatry, Oregon Health and Science University; and Associate Director for Education, Veterans Administration Northwest Network, Mental Illness Research, Education, and Clinical Center (MIRECC), Portland, Oregon

DANIEL J. CARLAT, MD, Editor-in-Chief, The Carlat Psychiatry Report; and Assistant Clinical Professor of Psychiatry, Tufts University School of Medicine, Boston, Massachusetts

MICHAEL K.S. CHENG, MD, FRCP(C), Mood and Anxiety Clinic, Children's Hospital of Eastern Ontario (CHEO); and University of Ottawa, Ottawa, Ontario, Canada

STEPHEN COLE, PhD, Training Institute for Suicide Assessment, Stoddard, New Hampshire

LISA B. DIXON, MD, MPH, VA Capitol Network (VISN 5) Mental Illness Research, Education, and Clinical Center (MIRECC), VA Maryland Healthcare System; and Professor, Department of Psychiatry, Division of Services Research, University of Maryland School of Medicine, Baltimore, Maryland

RON GREEN, MD, Training Institute for Suicide Assessment, Stoddard, New Hampshire

LESTON HAVENS, MD, Professor of Psychiatry, Harvard Medical School, Boston; and Cambridge Health Alliance, Cambridge, Massachusetts

ALLAN M. JOSEPHSON, MD, Division of Child and Adolescent Psychiatry, Department of Psychiatry and Behavioral Sciences, University of Louisville, Louisville, Kentucky

DAVID J. KNESPER, MD, Associate Professor of Psychiatry, Department of Psychiatry, University of Michigan Medical School; Director, Hospital and Community Psychiatry Section; and Director, Psychosomatic Medicine Program, University of Michigan Health System, Ann Arbor, Michigan

JACK KRASUSKI, MD, Executive Director, Blue Tower Institute LLC, Lyons, Illinois

GRACIANA LAPETINA, MD, Training Institute for Suicide Assessment, Stoddard, New Hampshire

JAMES MORRISON, MD, Professor of Clinical Psychiatry, Oregon Health and Science University, Portland, Oregon

AARON MURRAY-SWANK, PhD, VA Capitol Network (VISN 5) Mental Illness Research, Education, and Clinical Center (MIRECC), VA Maryland Healthcare System; and Assistant Professor, Department of Psychiatry, Division of Services Research, University of Maryland School of Medicine, Baltimore, Maryland

EKKEHARD OTHMER, MD, PhD, Adjunct Professor of Psychiatry, Department of Psychiatry, University of Kansas Medical Center, Kansas City, Kansas; and Medical Director, Picture Hills Psychiatric Center, Kansas City, Missouri

J. PHILIPP OTHMER, MD, Assistant Professor of Psychiatry, Department of Psychiatry, VA Medical Center, Kansas City, Missouri

SIEGLINDE C. OTHMER, PhD, Director, Picture Hills Psychiatric Center, Kansas City, Missouri

JOHN R. PETEET, MD, Department of Psychiatry, Harvard Medical School, Boston, Massachusetts

PHILLIP J. RESNICK, MD, Professor, Department of Psychiatry, Case Western Reserve, Cleveland, Ohio

DAVID J. ROBINSON, MD, FRCPC, FAPA, Associate Professor, Department of Psychiatry, London Health Sciences Center–South Street Hospital; and Faculty of Medicine and Dentistry, University of Western Ontario, London, Ontario, Canada

SHAWN CHRISTOPHER SHEA, MD, Director, Training Institute for Suicide Assessment and Clinical Interviewing, Stoddard; and Adjunct Assistant Professor of Psychiatry, Dartmouth Medical School, Hanover, New Hampshire

JOHN SOMMERS-FLANAGAN, PhD, Associate Professor of Counselor Education, Educational Leadership and Counseling, The University of Montana, Missoula, Montana

CONTRIBUTORS continued

RITA SOMMERS-FLANAGAN, PhD, Professor of Counselor Education, Educational Leadership and Counseling, The University of Montana, Missoula, Montana

BETTE STEWART, MS, Department of Psychiatry, Division of Services Research, University of Maryland School of Medicine, Baltimore, Maryland

Clinical Interviewing: Practical Tips from Master Clinicians

in the treatment of persons who have serious mental illness is widely recognized. This article provides a practical interviewing guide for mental health professionals who work with patients who have serious mental illness and their families. The article begins by considering the role of the family in the inpatient phase of treatment and then moves to a discussion of working with families while the consumer is in outpatient care.

Psychiatrists now recognize that religion and spirituality are important to much of the populace and that attending to them probably will improve clinical psychiatric practice. This article presents a practical guide for addressing some of the key interviewing skills needed to explore a patient's framework for meaning—the patient's religion, spirituality, and worldview. It offers guidelines on the process of the interview, including ways to initiate conversation in this area, with suggestions and specific questions for a more thorough exploration of the patient's religious and spiritual life.

The American Board of Psychiatry and Neurology Psychiatry Part II Examination (the "oral boards") is among the most challenging examinations in all of medicine. The pass rate for the oral boards has hovered around 55% to 60% for years and remains lower than in other medical specialties. This article is a primer on how to pass the oral bards. It is based on the author's experience of personally training more than 400 psychiatry oral board candidates each year.

The "Interviewing Tips of the Month" on the Website of the Training Institute for Suicide Assessment and Clinical Interviewing are supplied by visitors to the Website or by participants in the author's workshops.

Each month the author chooses a favorite tip for posting and then adds the past month's tip to the "Tip Archive." This article describes eight effective tips for uncovering sensitive material such as antisocial behavior, substance abuse, and physical violence as well as a technique for improving medication adherence.

This article presents specific tips for detecting malingering and the risk of violence. Specific topics include detailed inquiry into symptoms, endorsement of bogus symptoms, and confrontation of a patient with a paranoid persecutor. It ends with strategic tips and an illustrative dialogue showing how these tips can be implemented in practice.

A review of some practical interviewing techniques for assessing the presence of bipolar disorder and attention-deficit/hyperactivity disorder. Case studies and interview excerpts illustrate the key interviewing techniques.

This article provides practical tips for exploring delusions and substance abuse. Specific tips include "greasing the wheels for exploring delusions," "handling the question, 'Do you believe me?' with a delusional patient," and "obtaining a more accurate substance abuse history." It ends with a dialogue illustrating the use of these techniques.

Disengagement is the main enemy for the consultation-liaison psychiatrist. The goal of the first interview is to transform the unwilling, uncooperative, and often difficult and hostile patient into an engaged interview participant. Otherwise, the interview is an unproductive interrogation and an unpleasant power struggle. Once the difficult patient is engaged, the more typical psychiatric interview can begin. The three interview-engagement tips or techniques described are among the author's favorite ways to overcome the impediments to engagement most often associated with difficult patients.

@ Additional Material Available online.

FORTHCOMING ISSUES

RECENT ISSUES

THE CLINICS ARE NOW AVAILABLE ONLINE!

Access your subscription at:
http://www.theclinics.com

Preface

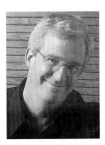

Shawn Christopher Shea, MD
Guest Editor

I t has been my experience over the years that too often words such as "unique" and "outstanding" find their ways into prefaces and introductions. In this instance, it may be justifiable to use them; I hope you will agree as you enjoy this issue of the *Psychiatric Clinics of North America*. Rather than give a one- or two-sentence synopsis of the articles (each author has provided a concise synopsis in the Table of Contents), the editor of the *Psychiatric Clinics*, Sarah Barth, suggested that in the Preface I say something about the unusual genesis of this issue that reflects its unique qualities.

Let me begin by saying that it is an honor to be guest editor of this issue of the *Psychiatric Clinics of North America*. I believe it is the first time in the history of psychiatry that any journal has chosen to devote an entire issue to the practical art of clinical interviewing, and it should be emphasized that this issue is about clinical interviewing, not its close cousin psychotherapy. Having had the privilege of studying interviewing for nearly 30 years, I can say that such an issue is, in my opinion, long overdue. At last, the complexities and nuances of the interviewing skills—that we all, as clinicians, know are the core of our healing art—have been given the attention they warrant in a highly respected journal. In this sense I think it may be safe to say that this issue is indeed unique.

I think this issue may be unique in yet another fashion. We wanted the articles to read with the informality of a valued clinician sharing his or her best clinical pearls, as if we were standing at the bedside of a patient on rounds or in a room with a trusted supervisor. Consequently, all the authors were asked to write their articles in an informal style using first person, exactly as they teach. Our collective goal as contributors was to create an easy-reading "book," one that we wish had been available to us during our residencies (and afterwards as

0193-953X/07/$ – see front matter
doi:10.1016/j.psc.2007.03.004

well), brimming with practical ideas and suggestions for overcoming everyday challenges written in an enjoyable and no-nonsense fashion.

The conception of the issue was unusual in another regard, also, because it is a spin-off from the Internet. Since 1999, I have had the opportunity of editing an on-line feature at the Training Institute for Suicide Assessment and Clinical Interviewing (www.suicideassessment.com) called the "Interviewing Tip of the Month." These interviewing tips are supplied, not by myself, but by visitors to the Website and participants from my workshops on clinical interviewing. At the time of this publication there are more than 85 such clinical gems archived on this Website.

I learned so much from these tips that it struck me, "What would happen if I asked the greatest interviewers of our time to provide two or three of their best tips each?" I originally had thought of posting these tips on the Website itself but subsequently was offered the rare opportunity to do so in the *Psychiatric Clinics of North America.* Consequently, in Part II, "Favorite Tips from Those Who Wrote the Book," you will find the favorite tips of some of your favorite authors covering an array of challenging interviewing tasks, from the assessment of violence and malingering to engaging difficult patients and uncovering psychotic process.

Here is where I feel the word "outstanding" can be legitimately applied, because I believe it is the first time that such a collection of interviewing experts—most of whom have, as the section title suggests, written the gold-standard books on clinical interviewing—has been assembled to provide their very best tips in a single publication, whether book or journal.

To round out the clinical thrust of the journal, there were certain particularly difficult aspects of clinical interviewing that I felt deserved a more detailed exploration. I collected these in Part I, "Innovative Strategies for Navigating Difficult Clinical Interviewing Tasks." Some topics, such as enhancing the therapeutic alliance, were chosen (despite having an extensive literature already devoted to them) because of their key importance and because innovative developments, such as "motivational interviewing," have opened new doorways to the art of engagement.

In contrast, other topics were chosen because so little had been written about them, despite their critical importance. Thus you will find splendid articles on how to talk with patients about their spirituality and worldview and how to engage and help the family members of those suffering from severe mental illnesses such as schizophrenia, bipolar disorder, and obsessive-compulsive disorder. These are the types of immediately practical articles that I think every psychiatric resident and mental health professional, across all disciplines, should read and savor for their wisdom. In addition I thought I would be remiss if I did not include an article on one of the difficult "clinical" tasks that we all must navigate, passing the oral boards. I believe the resulting article will prove to be a must-read for any newly minted clinician approaching this daunting rite-of-passage.

One more aspect of this issue of the *Psychiatric Clinics* may warrant the distinction of the word "unique." Although this is not a journal devoted to issues related to residency training and educational technology itself, the editors of the *Psychiatric Clinics* have agreed to include an entire section on topics of immediate importance to residency directors and supervisors. Part III, "Training Psychiatric Residents in Clinical Interviewing: State-of-the-Art Strategies for Residency Directors and Interviewing Mentors," focuses on practical issues related to the development of interviewing training courses and innovations in supervision such as macrotraining and facilic supervision. For nearly 20 years my friends and colleagues at the Department of Psychiatry at the Dartmouth Medical School have been vigorously pushing the envelope on methods of teaching clinical interviewing skills, and this set of four articles reflects their efforts.

Adding to this unique stance–creating an issue devoted to both the description of clinical interviewing skills and to the methods for teaching those skills–this issue of the *Psychiatric Clinics of North America*, which began with the Internet, ends with it as well. Three of the educational articles are to be found solely on the Web in our "Web archive." I would like to think that these lengthy "articles" are special, because, in essence, they are monographs regarding specific supervision techniques (including a programmed text on facilic supervision that can be downloaded and given by supervisors to their psychiatric residents). Because of their length, they never would have been amenable to publication in a standard journal format, but Sarah Barth at the *Psychiatric Clinics* (to whom I owe a debt of gratitude) had the creativity to suggest placing them on the Web, where enough space could be devoted to the supervision techniques to make them come to life for supervisors.

Finally, I would like to thank all the authors for their time and wisdom. As with all issues of the *Psychiatric Clinics*, the authors are the cream of the crop. We could not have hoped for a more impressive group of master clinicians. It has been a privilege to work and to learn from all of them. In particular, I should like to thank Dr. Leston Havens, whose writings inspired and guided me back when I was a psychiatric resident in the early 1980s. I have always hoped to have the honor of being involved in a project of which Dr. Havens was a part. His wonderful article leads off our issue, and, as usual, he has produced an article at once both provocative and wonderfully practical. Enjoy!

Shawn Christopher Shea, MD

E-mail address: sheainte@worldpath.net

Part I

Innovative Strategies for Navigating Difficult

Clinical Interviewing Tasks

Approaching the Mind in Clinical Interviewing: The Techniques of Soundings and Counterprojection

Leston Havens, MD[a,b,*]

[a]Harvard Medical School, 25 Shattuck Street, Boston, MA 02115, USA
[b]Cambridge Health Alliance, 1493 Cambridge Street, Cambridge, MA 02139, USA

It is with great pleasure that I have the opportunity to write the lead article in this unusual and highly practical issue of the *Psychiatric Clinics of North America*, in which the focus is solely upon the art, craft, and science of clinical interviewing. It is a particular honor for I feel that, for the first time in the history of psychiatry and psychology, many of the great innovators in clinical interviewing have been assembled into one volume, each providing their favorite interviewing tips and unique perspectives.

As the lead article I decided to emphasize a point, strongly shared by the editor of this issue, Dr. Shea [1], that all interviewing is enhanced by an understanding of the psychodynamics in which it invariably unfolds. I am hoping that this article will set a perspective from which the wonderful articles that follow can be more powerfully understood and their techniques more effectively employed.

In particular, I hope that my emphasis on the psychodynamic interplay of the interviewer and the interviewee will accomplish two things: first, that it will provide an integrating model with which to assimilate all of the wisdom that follows in the subsequent articles; second, that it will show how an understanding of psychodynamics can move directly from theory to practice by illustrating two specific interviewing techniques–soundings and counterprojection–that derive directly from psychodynamic understanding.

THE INITIAL INTERVIEW: THE PLACE IN WHICH TWO MINDS MEET

When an interviewer and a patient meet, it is the meeting place of two minds. Both minds directly affect the other through conscious statements; both minds

*Cambridge Health Alliance, 1493 Cambridge Street, Cambridge, MA 02139. *E-mail address*: sgallant@challiance.org

0193-953X/07/$ – see front matter
doi:10.1016/j.psc.2007.02.005
psych.theclinics.com

indirectly affect the other through unconscious processes; both minds will forever be changed. There is no other way. At the end of the initial interview, two slightly different people emerge from the office, whether they are aware of this fact or not.

An initial interview is essentially a delightful stew in which the unconscious minds of two people intertwine and stir about in the mysterious nuances of each other's shadows. To understand this process I believe it is best to begin by better conceptualizing what is meant by the "mind."

In psychiatry, from a historical perspective, the mind was often viewed, rather awkwardly, as if it could be conceptualized like the brain, essentially functioning as a container of thoughts as the brain was a container of neurons. What if the mind is not simply a container to be reached into and sampled, as we say, something self-contained? And what if this static neurologic metaphor has become an outdated model of the brain itself? How are we then to describe mind? In particular, how are the contemporary clinical interviewer and therapist to imagine it today?

These are not idle or merely academic questions, because the way we imagine mind affects how we approach it, and, subsequently, how we approach the initial interview. If we see mind as a closed container to be reached into, we risk doing solely just that, as witnessed by the questions and probings of descriptive psychiatry and of examining physicians in other branches of medicine.

Psychiatrists, as trained physicians, long schooled in the ways of the physical examination of the body, sometimes tend to approach the mind as if it were merely a piece of the body. They want the mind to stand still, as the body may stand still while it is investigated. They want the mind to cooperate, answer, even testify against itself. Most important, the mind in this view can be studied without essentially changing it. Reflexes can be tested, blood drawn off, even parts of the body removed for study, without changing significantly the state of body or, by implication, of the mind.

From an analytic perspective, which is more subtle, the clinician still may see the mind as a container or as being divided into subcontainers. With different degrees of accessibility, we may question one subcontainer, with another be patient asking only for associations, and be even more patient with a third subcontainer of the mind, waiting on those perhaps deeper revelations of self—transferences—to crystallize before us.

Clearly, these views of the mind, which stem directly from a longstanding comparison with the brain, have become outdated, because their model, the brain itself, is far less static and stable as once thought. For most of the twentieth century, the brain seemed to be an early-maturing, fixed structure difficult to relate to the mind. The brain was a stable structure, constructing few new cells and presenting itself as largely unchanged through much of life. No wonder that a fluid mind envisioned as based on a static brain seemed to be an uneasy metaphor, because, at a basic level, the two seemed to be worlds apart.

Today, the metaphor works better for we are aware that the brain, like the mind, is shaped partly by experience. There are no containers and subcontainers in the brain. One cannot cleanly define where the sensory system ends and the motor system begins, because they are entwined and interlocked. Moreover, they are not static. They change. We now know that, even in adults, synapses constantly are being built, torn down, and new ones rebuilt. This newly understood neuroplasticity unites brain and mind in their shared characteristic of ever-evolving flux. The Nobel prizes given for brain research celebrated some of the ways the brain reflects its experience [2–3]. Perhaps as we come to understand the brain, it will seem more and more like mind, subtle, responsive, and, most of all, difficult to locate.

Now that from the perspective of a more modern neurophysiology, we can see that the mind and the brain may indeed have much in common, let us return to our pressing question: what exactly do we mean by mind? In particular, what are the properties of the mind that an interviewer meets or may fail to meet as the participants in an initial interview sit down together?

The interviewer's account cannot be wholly introspective or dependent on cognitive tests (eg, of the strength or brightness of mind) or on the mind as revealed by its products (eg, the judgments of art, literature, and science). The interviewer's goals are different from those of the art critic. Clinicians are not there solely to observe and absorb: we are there to seek out what is hidden and to heal what is difficult to find. The goal of the interviewer is transformation guided by compassion, not simply critique.

THE INVASIVE PROPERTY OF MIND

Very quickly in Freud's therapeutic work direct methods of approaching mind gave way to indirect ones because he concluded that the most important parts of mind were not the ones most accessible. Paradoxically, however, he also noted that what seemed to him the most important property of mind therapeutically was difficult to access, because it was at once both active and potentially invasive. The patient's unconscious could reach out and touch the unconscious of the interviewer, and often did so. The patient related personally to the clinician, and this relating connected the patient both to outwardly recognizable features of the therapist and to faint or even absent features of the therapist that the patient nevertheless imagined were present (ie, transference). Therapists themselves were changed by this relating/distorting property: they could come to feel and think and act as if they were what the patient imagined, a truly dynamic mixing of the unconscious! Let us look at an example:

> A brilliant, attractive patient excited in her therapist the feeling he must somehow possess or even enslave her. This was the way her mother had acted and both her husbands. With the mother and the first husband the patient experienced a growing wariness and eventually escaped. As the therapist acknowledged his feelings toward the patient, the patient grew bolder and was able to reduce the second husband's possessiveness and create a livable relationship.

In short, some of the most important parts of the mind are not only buried or unconscious; in Freud's view; they also can emerge and attach themselves to and affect the therapist. In doing so they are no longer unconscious, because the patient sees them, often literally, in the person of the therapist. They do remain unconscious in a different sense; the patient sees them but does not know that he or she has created them. The patient is unconscious that they are partly his or her own. The mind is capable of appearing and its ownership going unrecognized, being present and absent at once. It is as if mind were the product of a supremely absent-minded author, an author also capable of cribbing products from earlier needs and experiences and committing unconscious plagiarism on an enormous scale. This plagiarism or transference cannot always be easily confronted or corrected.

The capacity to create and recreate worlds, whether authored by the patient, the clinician or both parties, is imagination. It is through imagination that we can flee. But it is also by imagination that we can go in search. It is both a wondrous and necessary tool of the interviewer.

CLINICAL IMAGINATION IN THE INITIAL INTERVIEW

By clinical imagination I mean the delicate uncovering, sometimes objective and more often subjective, of the possible interweavings of patients' biologic vicissitudes, their unconscious processes, and their life experiences, all of which interviewers must discover to understand their patients. The information is most detailed, precise, and objective about the body. Frequently, a considerable number of unconscious possibilities also can be pinned down.

Curiously, the least systematic and detailed knowledge often concerns the patient's internal experience of the world as it is unfolding in real time: what happens and how it feels as it happens. The interviewer must plumb not only the unconscious phenomena possibly underlying changes in mood or behavior, but also what exactly happened and then how the report of what happened is told to the clinician, frequently distorted by the patient's internal experience of the world. What are the principal events that befall a 17-year-old going off to college or a woman with a wandering husband? What is the "real" that the interviewer should imagine?

Truth be told, however much people are ruled by biologic and unconscious processes, they live in their recalled experience of the "actual" and first must be met there, no matter how much their "actual" experience is a distortion of the real. Successful therapeutic meeting depends on the ability to make a projection into the experience of the other, that is, in Buber's [4] phrase, "to imagine the real."

Our imaginative investigations can fail secondary to a broad range of clinical gremlins. On the one hand, the patient may not internally "exist"; he or she may not "be" anywhere; the mind or self or person may be psychologically lost. Or the patient may barely exist, as when people live, as we say, from "mouth to mouth"; they wait on the words of others, tending to agree with and imitate whomever they are with, a perpetual disappearance of the real self. In such instances, because there is nothing inside the patient, the interviewer may mistakenly find himself or herself in the patient; the empty patient functions as a mirror. Unhappily, these "hollow men" are common and can be easily overlooked or misunderstood. Even more problematic, a clinician plagued by more than a fair share of narcissistic needs may be delighted to find himself or herself in the mirror provided by the patient. Pathology begets more pathology, and no one is healed.

Such shallow existences, which can directly cause our imaginative explorations to be absolutely wrong if we are not aware of this potential hazard in the initial interview, can come in many flavors. Children sometimes lose their existence between warring parents and themselves are only this side and that side of the quarrels. Actors, too, may exist in their parts and be empty or bewildered offstage. Others exist in a transcendental world of unlimited hopes and fancies; none of the realities of life touch them. Still others you cannot find at all: you may see a brilliant smile or the trace of an expression, but their speech dissolves, and they seem affectless when you approach; it is like looking into a hole. Existential psychiatry constructs its pathology out of the differing types and amounts of this nonexistence.

There are also people who exist but are so deeply hidden that they defeat every effort to locate them. They may, on the other hand, be so exquisitely sensitive and uncertain that they transform as soon as they are seen. Like chameleons, they change and disappear into the background colors of their wildly rich worlds. Sometimes, too, these hidden, changing, reflective existences function as masks, tricking the initial interviewer into thinking he or she has seen the actor when only the role was in the room. This is the nature of our psychologic work as psychiatrists, psychologists, counselors, and therapists: we can seldom be sure either that we have found the real person or if there is a person at all.

Thus far we have seen the roadblocks to the accurate projections of our imaginations, which are caused directly by the patient. A failure in imaginative inquiry also may arise from the therapist.

He or she may be unwilling or unable to imagine the actual internal world of the other. Sometimes there are good clinical reasons not to do so. It can be dangerous to get close to some people. Many paranoid patients, for example, have been so victimized by their actual experiences of closeness that they deal violently with too rapid an approach.

Our failures also can spring from a very well-intentioned effort to be well-informed. Many clinicians become like the White Knight in *Alice in Wonderland*. Their clinical imaginations are so stocked that they can hardly move at all. Every time the White Knight took a step, something fell off—a bucket, a sword, or a saucer. The White Knight knew he had a long way to go on his quest; he had wanted to be ready; but he had no backpack to keep things compartmentalized effectively. Many medical students, psychiatric residents, clinical psychology interns, and counseling interns feel this way. In some respects, it is an expected right of passage for all clinicians who appropriately push themselves toward excellence. In the early years of training, and sometimes much later as well, everything the patient says or does sets in motion so many trains of thought, so many possibilities, that the clinician is afraid to hear any more lest he or she forget something. At such moments there is no finding the patient, nor even ourselves.

Clinical imagination must be carried lightly, and it must be brought lightly to the patient, because, as we have just seen, there are many ways it can go astray. Everyone recognizes those who come on too strong. Empathy may be the imaginative projection of oneself into the mind of the other, but it does not mean the substitution of oneself for the other; in fact, it means the temporary setting aside of oneself for the other, perhaps the supreme psychologic asceticism. Nevertheless, the most empathic therapist in the world does not himself or herself go out of existence. If he or she succeeds in being Carl Rogers' [5] pane of glass through which the patient can be seen, that pane of glass is cloudy. The question now becomes: are there ways to make the glass more clear, to improve the accuracy of our imaginative explorations?

SOUNDINGS: MORE ACCURATELY GAUGING THE DEPTH OF A PATIENT'S FEELINGS AND INTENTIONS

This interviewing strategy–soundings–drew its name and its methodology from a most unexpected "clinician," Samuel Clemens, or Mark Twain as he is more commonly known. He drew his pen name from the process that riverboat captains used to discover the depth of the treacherous Mississippi River.

In unknown waters, a leadsman would throw over a weighted rope until it hit bottom and then call up the depth as indicated by the length of rope, yelling out a phrase such as, "By the mark four!" or "Mark three-and-one-half!" If the depth was found to be 2 fathoms, the boat was in danger of going aground, and the leadsman would urgently call out, "Mark twain!" Such a process was called "soundings" [6]. It was an accurate way of seeing what could not be seen–the bottom of the river. Years ago, I became interested in the idea that a similar interview strategy could be used to discern patients' hidden thoughts and intentions more accurately, even at the first meeting.

With soundings, the interviewer tosses out specific statements and watches how the patient responds to them. The responses often represent a fairly accurate record of how much the patient agrees or disagrees with the statement proffered by the clinician. With each "sounding," like our riverboat men, we get a more accurate feeling for what is hidden.

I believe this strategy will be understood more easily by way of an example. Let us take a look at a common clinical conundrum–trying to determine accurately a patient's intention to do something, perhaps leave an abusive marriage. Watch as the clinician, in this prototypic conversation helps both the patient and herself ferret out the patient's intention. The patient announces that she intends to leave her husband soon. What does this statement really mean?

How much intention is behind this statement? The interviewer tosses out a series of soundings to see where the depth of the intention actually lies:

> Patient: I really feel that somehow I need to get out of this relationship. I know in my heart, Jim is bad for me. I'll get out soon.
> Clinician: You dream of this?
> Patient: As a matter of fact, I think of it every day. I know that Jim is perhaps my biggest problem.
> Clinician: You might want to do this then, to leave?
> Patient: Yea, I might need to do it.
> Clinician: You feel you can do it?
> Patient [sighs]: Well, I guess so . . . I think so.
> Clinician: You feel you will do it within a month or two?
> Patient: Well, I doubt that. . . . No I don't think that is in the cards in the near future.

Watch the technique at use in another tricky clinical situation, determining the degree to which a patient believes in a delusion. Perhaps a patient presents in an emergency room with a delusion that he is being constantly watched. The following series of soundings can help the clinician decide the level of conviction the patient has regarding his delusion, a concept sometimes called the "distance" a patient has from a delusion: "You may wonder can this be true?"; "There's too much evidence to doubt it?"; "There doesn't seem any doubt at all?" The clinician pauses after each of these soundings to see how the patient responds.

In evaluating the level of the patient's intention to act on the delusion, the following soundings might be of use, once again with a pause after each one to listen to the patient's response: "You've thought of doing something about it?"; "You want to do something about it?"; and "You've planned to do something about it?"

Perhaps one of the most powerful arenas for using soundings is in the attempt to uncover accurately a patient's intention of acting upon suicidal ideation. The gateway to this use of soundings is the sophisticated use of empathic statements. Empathic statements, a basic clinical tool, are remarks intended to imitate, acknowledge, share, or deepen a patient's feeling state. These statements range from exclamations ("How awful!"; "How frightening!") through simple statements ("You must be terrified") to more complex forms ("No wonder you feel terrified!"). Empathic statements place the observer close to and able to share the patient's feelings or memory states. They also, intrinsically, are testing methods, that is, soundings. Because we can never do more than approximate what another person is feeling or remembering, the nature of the other's response to our empathic statement provides data on how accurate our approximation has been. It is here that empathic statements can play a powerful role in suicide assessment.

In evaluating suicidal intent, a succession of empathic remarks tests the level of the suicidality the person has reached. "You may feel awful" or "This may be more than you can bear" sounds a level of general distress. "You may want to die," "You do want to die," and "You have planned out how to die" plumb increasingly dangerous levels of intent. I like to call this level of succession "going below." The purpose is to establish how far down the patient follows. Often, part way down, the patient corrects a statement and perhaps remembers some happy event that has improved his or her mood. Other patients fall all the way to the bottom, which puts the observer in touch with the extremity of their pain.

The strategy of soundings can be used in many difficult clinical situations. It is a nice way of using intuition and imagination to gain a more accurate reading of the patient's internal experience. Interviewing technique, in this instance, allows us to sharpen the image that our imaginations create in the clinical interview, decreasing the distortions that occur when two minds meet.

PSYCHOLOGIC SAFETY: THE IMPORTANCE OF FINDING A WORKING DISTANCE

Besides the previously mentioned problems associated with the distortions at work, as we try to use our imaginations effectively to understand the inner experiences of the patient, another critical clinical issue quickly emerges in an initial interview: safety. Does the patient feel psychologically safe in the room with the interviewer, and does the interviewer feel safe with the patient? It is frightening to see a clinician for the first time, to open one's soul to a total stranger. One patient put it brilliantly when she commented that there is always the possibility of a "mind rape."

Keeping these concerns in mind, the initial interviewer walks a fine line attempting to be close enough to find the other but not so close as to smother the other so that all therapeutic independence is lost or to frighten the other so that no second session occurs. Many have remarked on what a curious and vexing combination of closeness and distance both clinical interviewing and psychotherapy represent.

Winnicott [7] introduced the idea of being alone with another. He meant that it is possible to sit near someone in an interview room, for example, and be or not be alone. This is a pre-eminently psychological idea, because what "close" means here is not bodily presence or absence but the subjective experience of feeling invaded, needing to please, or in some other way being pulled out of shape by the presence of another. Winnicott is indirectly addressing the issue of safety. Not being able to be alone with someone is to lack self-possession in that person's presence.

Of course most of our boundaries, which provide a sense of psychological safety, become tenuous in the presence of the very beautiful, the very rich, or the very famous and when we are in love. In such circumstances, however much we want "to keep our head," it is all too human to "sell out" or find ourselves doing foolish things. Sometimes even defiance is a defensive response to the presence of powerful or potentially alluring figures. But the response I want to discuss, however, is almost the opposite of defiance: empathy–a sense of merging with and losing ourselves in the other.

The therapist is to be present to listen empathically (and perhaps even gently encourage the faint rumblings of the patient's real self–as opposed to the social self–as it begins warily to emerge in the interview) yet, simultaneously, and most importantly, not to invade. Hence Freud recommended an "evenly-suspended attention." Note what this says about distance and closeness in the interview. The therapist needs to be psychologically very close to catch the faint signals from the wary patient and very distant so as not to distort them: a curious and vexing combination indeed! An example from ongoing therapy can highlight this paradoxical process:

> A much-admired patient induced in his therapist a fear of displeasing the patient by letting him down. It was important to tell the patient of both the admiration and the fear. Doing so relieved the therapist's self-consciousness and expressed to the shy patient the extent of the therapist's admiration. Closeness and distance were then both present to the patient at the same moment and in a way that remained memorable.

I believe it is the acknowledgment of this paradox that brings interpersonal considerations strongly into focus in both the initial interview and in ongoing psychotherapy, as well as in therapeutic relationships that focus primarily on psychopharmacology. If we meet, we must sometimes collide. Unless we are unwilling to deal with these collisions, we cannot be set too far apart from each other. What we need to find is a principle that allows us to become close with our patients while mediating the inevitable conflicts that such closeness begets. I call this Bromberg's "common property principle": whatever occurs in the intersubjective space, which is the psychological meeting ground of the patient and the therapist, is the common property of both [8]. Both participants must feel safe within this common psychological space for the interview to proceed smoothly.

To secure this safe space, there is one thing we must be willing to do, and as clinicians we must become talented at doing–negotiate. Gifted interviewers are gifted negotiators of psychological space, rules, and agreements. To negotiate gracefully as clinicians, we must be willing to acknowledge both our invasiveness and the possibility of our being wrong. When appropriate we also must be able to apologize. The common property principle says that whatever occurs in the intersubjective space belongs to both of us. We cannot remove it as "just ours" or disown it by blaming the other. We must live it and negotiate it together.

But how do we take these intriguing, albeit highly intellectual considerations, and transform them into a useful interviewing technique that can help us help our patients feel safe in the initial interview?

FROM THEORY TO PRACTICE: THE ART OF COUNTERPROJECTION

For a moment, let us look at patients who are wary or perhaps even paranoid. When first meeting us, such patients expect trouble. They do not feel safe. They anticipate invasion of their psychological space by us, and they commonly project out their own wariness and anger onto us, at which point the interview relationship may already be lost.

From the perspective of Bromberg's principle, there is no common space. The patient has his or her own space and sees us as sitting in our own space, and fears that we intend to invade. There is no common ground. Such paranoid patients are traditionally some of the most difficult people to engage. Second appointments are rarities.

Harry Stack Sullivan, one of the most gifted interviewers of all time, had a variety of clever ways of creating shared space with such patients, a sense of being with them as opposed to being against them. It is worthwhile to take a look at his work for a moment, because it offers the beginnings of the counterprojective technique that I have found so valuable over the years and that I hope will prove to be of value to you.

Sullivan's intuitive understanding of the approach to shy, suspicious, or angry people foreshadows couterprojection. He suggested sitting beside or at an angle to the patient, to avoid staring at self-conscious people and also to direct attention somewhere else—out there. This "out there" is a commonly shared space that both the interviewer and the interviewee look at together. In essence, the "bad guys" are out there somewhere, not in this room.

This "out there" or somewhere else is society itself, which in Sullivan's framework is where a lot of real psychopathology originated or is enabled. For patients, it feels remarkably safer to experience the bad guy as "out there," not as the therapist sitting in the room with them. Redirecting clinical attention away from the interviewing dyad nonverbally moves the "projective screen" away from the therapist, where it can do damage. The question is, are there verbal techniques that can even more effectively create Bromberg's common property?

When I first described counterprojection in an article many years ago, I found the following everyday illustration of people responding to acute pain to be useful in introducing the power of the technique [9]. For example, badly stubbing one's toe on a loose brick typically results in anger toward the brick, blaming of it, even the desire to kick the offending object again. A friend who tries to add solace by comforting the fallen person (perhaps even touching the injured friend) is sometimes shunned away because of overstimulation, almost as if there is a transference of anger towards the friend meant to be directed at the brick. Moreover, the hurt person may resent questioning, sometimes implying that the friend should already know what the matter is, suggesting a temporary loss of ego boundaries.

On the other hand there is one thing the friend can do that will not bother the injured person at all: pick up the brick and throw it, yelling, "That damn brick!" Just such an exclamation against a "common enemy" is a prototypic form of counterprojective speech. Just as Sullivan nonverbally creates a common "out there" where the "bad guys" are by his seating arrangement, the friend has, through the verbal phrase "That damn brick!" created an "out there" by attacking the "bad guy," which happens to be an inanimate brick in this instance. It is very hard for someone to be mad at someone else who is attacking a common enemy.

In counterprojection the interviewer counters (deflects) a patient's projection by pointing attention away from himself or herself and toward another object.

A counterprojective statement has three components. First, it must point "out there," because in part projection follows attention. Second, it must speak specifically about the figures being projected; counterprojective statements place the brick, boss, girlfriend, or parent on the projective screen before the therapist and patient. Perhaps "speak about" is not right. No interpretation or explanation concerning these figures is offered; that would invite discussion centered back again on therapist and patient; the figures are simply put "out there." Third, in order to move projections, some part of the patient's negative feelings about those figures must be jointly expressed by the therapist.

Counterprojection is a gentle technique. One must be careful not to attack a specific person verbally in such a way that it inflames the patient's anger toward that person. Rather, the comments are made as temporary points of understanding of the patient's viewpoint and generally are phrased in the third person, such as, "He always seems interested in himself," or "They never seem to see your side of things clearly." Sometimes society itself is the aim of counterprojection: "It's rough out there now"; "Times are so tough, a good man can't make a reasonable living out there"; or "Nobody seems to understand you."

In the following dialogue, a patient who is quite frustrated with his family, boss, and friends begins to get angry at the clinician for not providing answers. Note how the clinician deftly points away from himself (thus deflecting the patient's anger) using counterprojective statements that also convey a sense of empathy:

Patient: Why don't you clarify this? You know me very well, I'm confused.
Clinician: I agree, it is confusing.
Patient: I can't do this alone, you know.
Clinician: Neither your boss nor your girlfriend has clarified things either.
Patient: They haven't.
Clinician: Everywhere you look, no one helps [said empathically].
Patient: But you are supposed too.
Clinician: I suppose your parents were supposed to help, too.
Patient: They didn't [patient looks sad].
Clinician: No wonder you want someone out there to take their place. They left such a hole!

The clinician has deflected the patient's anger gracefully, provided a bit of insight, and now has opened the door to continue a conversation about the parents, effectively keeping the anger off of himself.

SUMMARY

The main premise of this article is that minds are fluid: when an interviewer and a patient meet, their minds meet and interact with each other. To be an effective interviewer, it is critical to understand the clinical gremlins that arise psychodynamically when these two minds interact. It is from an understanding of these psychodynamics that sound interviewing techniques can be designed to transform these gremlins.

I demonstrated that one of the main interactions of mind that occurs is the clinician's attempt to use his or her mind to enter imaginatively the patient's world of experience. Unfortunately this imaginative attempt to understand the patient's inner world of experience accurately can be thwarted by a variety of distorting mechanisms including the inability to see the patient's real self because of its defensive flight behind all sorts of unconscious and conscious masks. We then saw how our psychodynamic understanding of this problem led us to search for an interviewing technique—soundings—that can specifically enhance the ability of our imaginative forays to come back with more valid pictures of the real patient.

We also saw that a second major interaction between the minds of the interviewer and the patient is the joint process of finding interpersonal safety. From a psychodynamic perspective, finding a common ground, or common property as Bromberg puts it, can open the way to a psychologically safe environment.

We then looked at one of the most challenging arenas for establishing safety, paranoia, and found a specific interviewing technique based upon our psychodynamic understanding of the problem, counterprojection, that can help transform this thorny problem. Once again our main point is highlighted; a sound understanding of psychodynamics leads to the development of sound interviewing strategies and techniques.

In this article we have looked at just two complexities of the interviewing process and two solutions. In the following articles you are in for a treat, for some of the greatest interviewers in our field will explore numerous everyday interviewing traps and problems, providing concrete and immensely practical interviewing techniques for side-stepping those traps and solving those problems that are bound to occur when two minds meet.

References

[1] Shea SC. Psychiatric interviewing: the art of understanding. 2nd edition. Philadelphia: W.B. Saunders Company; 1998.

[2] Hubel, Sperry, Weisel, 1981.

[3] Carlsson, Greengard, Kandel, 2002.

[4] Buber M. Guilt and guilt feelings. In: Friedman M, editor. The knowledge of man. New York: Harper and Row; 1965.

[5] Rogers C. Client-centered therapy: its current practice, implications and theory. Boston: Houghton Mifflin; 1951.

[6] Welland D. The life and times of Mark Twain. New York: Crescent Books; 1991.

[7] Winnicott DW. The maturational process and the facilitating environment. New York: International Universities Press; 1965.

[8] Bromberg P. Standing in the spaces. Hillsdale (NJ): The Analytic Press; 1998.

[9] Havens LL. Explorations in the uses of language in psychotherapy: counterprojections. Contemp Psychoanal 1980;16:53–67.

New Approaches for Creating the Therapeutic Alliance: Solution-Focused Interviewing, Motivational Interviewing, and the Medication Interest Model

Michael K.S. Cheng, MD, FRCP(C)[a,b,*]

[a]Mood and Anxiety Clinic, Children's Hospital of Eastern Ontario (CHEO),
401 Smyth Road, Ottawa, Ontario, Canada K1H 8L1
[b]University of Ottawa, Ottawa, Ontario, Canada

P robably one of the most important skills learned as a medical student and as a psychiatry resident is building the therapeutic alliance. Knowing how to navigate the tricky complexities and subtle nuances of establishing a therapeutic alliance—especially in the initial encounter—is, arguably, the most critical skill clinicians possess, whether seeing a patient for a single interview or for long-term therapy.

As a trainee, I struggled however, because although there are literally thousands of research articles about the alliance and clinical interviewing, there are many fewer that focus on how exactly to form the alliance. In this article we will review the theory behind the therapeutic alliance and, more importantly, explores three new approaches to establishing it effectively: (1) solution-focused interviewing, (2) motivational interviewing, and (3) the medication interest model.

DEFINING THE THERAPEUTIC ALLIANCE

Research studies and common sense indicate that a good therapeutic alliance is essential for positive patient encounters and outcomes. Exactly what is this therapeutic alliance? Decades ago, Bordin [1] presented his ground-breaking transtheoretical conceptualization, in which he defined the alliance as having three main components:

- Agreement on goals, which are the desired outcomes of the therapeutic process
- Agreement on tasks, which are the steps that will be undertaken to achieve the goals

*Children's Hospital of Eastern Ontario (CHEO), 401 Smyth Road, Ottawa, Ontario, Canada K1H 8L1. E-mail address: www.drcheng.ca

0193-953X/07/$ – see front matter
doi:10.1016/j.psc.2007.01.003

- Bond between client and therapist, which encompasses Rogerian aspects such as trust, respect, genuineness, unconditional positive regard, and empathy.

WHAT IS THE MOST IMPORTANT FACTOR IN ESTABLISHING THE THERAPEUTIC ALLIANCE?

Most individuals would state that the most important factors for achieving a sound therapeutic alliance are listening to patients sensitively, being empathetic, and building trust and respect. Are these traditional factors really the most important?

Consider a very significant alliance–the alliance between the Allies during the Second World War. During that time, members of the alliance included the United States, Britain, Canada, and Russia. Was the alliance between Russia and the United States based on trust, respect, and empathy for one another? Probably not! The alliance was based more on mutual goals–the destruction of a common enemy.

Indeed, there is nothing wrong with having a relationship founded on mutual trust and empathy, but unfortunately in many situations the psychiatrist and the client will not yet have developed that sense of trust and empathy. For example, the psychiatrist might have just met the patient, or the patient might place a higher value on his or her autonomy than on bonding with the psychiatrist (like most teenaged patients!).

Fortunately, in addition to the traditional ways of securing the alliance through empathy, some exciting new strategies are available. These strategies focus on the power inherent in joining with the patient in a collaborative effort to define the goals and tasks defined by Bordin [1].

GOALS

What exactly are the goals Bordin [1] mentions in his first step in establishing an alliance? Goals are the intended outcome from the client–clinician interaction. Universal, normal goals for most people include

- Biologic needs such as food, shelter, safety, and physical health
- Various psychosocial needs such as being emotionally and psychologically well. These include needs for agency and autonomy (the desire to have a sense of competency or control in one's life) and affiliation (the need to have some sense of attention, connection, and relationship with other people).
- Spiritual needs, such as the quest for a sense of hope or meaning in one's life

Goals may vary with the individual's interpersonal style. For example, some individuals place a higher value on autonomy and agency, whereas others may place more value on affiliation and connection.

Goals also may vary across the life span. For example, adolescents typically have a higher need for autonomy and independence from adults, combined with an increased need to affiliate and connect with their peers.

Having identified the goals, the psychiatrist needs to understand how to achieve them–the second step in Bordin's [1] conceptualization.

TASKS

Tasks are what the patient (or therapist) does that moves the client toward healthy, therapeutic goals. Examples of physical tasks include ensuring good sleep, nutrition, exercise, and appropriate use of medications. Examples of psychotherapeutic tasks include identifying automatic thoughts and cognitive distortions (as in cognitive-behavior therapy), linking mood to interpersonal events (as in interpersonal psychotherapy), using solution-directed rather than problem-talk (as in solution-focused therapy), and instillation of hope (as in a common-factors approach). Examples of spiritual tasks include prayer or participating in a religious community.

Several points worth keeping in mind when setting goals and tasks. One should remember the crucial role of obtaining genuine, nonpressured agreement from the client on specific goals and the tasks chosen to achieve them. The clinician also should keep in mind how the strategic use of different tasks may help the patient achieve a single goal (eg, a relaxed state of mind may be achieved by using a variety of tasks: listening to gentle music, relaxation therapy, and the use of antianxiety agents). Although discussions tend to make a theoretical distinction between goals and tasks, such distinctions often blur together in clinical practice.

THE PRIMARY IMPORTANCE OF UNCOVERING THE PATIENT'S GOALS

Finding agreement on goals starts with finding out what the patient's goals actually are as opposed to what the clinician may think they should be. Although there are two main ways to interview clients (problem-based interviewing versus goal-based interviewing), only goal-based interviewing really asks about goals directly from the client's viewpoint.

Medical students typically are taught to start patient encounters by asking the classic, problem-based question: "What [problem] brings you in today?" and "What's been bothering you?" These questions usually lead the patient to answer in a narrative that moves from the past to the present.

For example, the patient may state, "I hurt my foot yesterday and today I can't walk on it anymore." After eliciting the problem, the clinician diagnoses the problem and determines the appropriate treatment to reach that goal. In most cases, the patient agrees. For example, the clinician may state, "You've broken your toe. You'll need to use crutches for the next several weeks, but the good news is that it will heal without your requiring a cast."

With straightforward medical conditions, goals are deduced easily, rendering it unnecessary actually to ask about goals. In fact, using goal-focused questions in such situations could sound quite silly, leading a patient to doubt the clinician's competence. For example:

> Patient: "I hurt my foot yesterday and today I can't walk on it anymore."
> Clinician: "So what would you like to get from coming here today?"
> Patient: "Isn't that obvious? Just fix my foot!"

When the situations or goals are not so obvious, however, problems can arise from relying solely on problem-based questioning. The following example shows the inherent traps with traditional problem-based interviewing when used with a reluctant teenager brought in by his parents:

Clinician: "What seems to be the problem?"
Teenager: "I don't have a problem. I don't need to be here. My parents need help, not me."
Clinician: "Your parents told me that your mood is irritable, you've lost interest in things, and you have trouble with your sleep, appetite, and concentration. Sounds to me like you might have a depression and need treatment for it."
Teenager: "I knew this was gonna be a waste of my time. I'm getting out of here!"

In this example, the alliance got off to a poor start, because the clinician and patient did not agree on goals; in addition, the clinician prematurely recommended treatment (ie, a task) before achieving a buy-in from the teenager on what the goals should be in the first place.

It also is interesting to note the meta-assumption posed by the question, "What problem brings you here?" The message to the patient seems to be, "You have a problem." Interestingly, "What's your problem?" (said in a sarcastic tone) is a common insult among teenagers. It is ironic how a simple problem-based question can end up being interpreted as an insult!

SOLUTION-FOCUSED INTERVIEWING: THE NEW WAVE IN ENGAGEMENT

In the 1990s a particularly innovative style of psychotherapy evolved that had many ramifications for establishing the therapeutic alliance more effectively in psychotherapy in general and in the initial interview as well. Solution-focused interviewing is a form of goal-directed interviewing. When the patient's goals cannot be assumed readily, I think that you will find that solution-focused interviewing can be exquisitely effective. Typical situations include chronic medical conditions and emotional, behavioral, or psychiatric problems. Solution-focused questions, with their ability to create hope and promote client strengths, figure prominently in ongoing solution-focused therapy [2–5]. Examples of solution-focused questions include

- "What would make this a helpful visit?"
- "What would you like to see different from coming here?"

The following example illustrates some of the advantages of solution-focused questions, revisiting the disgruntled teenager met earlier:

Clinician: "What's the problem that brings you here today?"
Teenager: "I don't have a problem. I don't need to be here. My parents need help, not me."
Clinician: "Okay—so what would make this a helpful visit?"

> Teenager: "Tell my parents that I don't need to be here; they're the ones who have the problem."
>
> Clinician: "Things sound stressful with your parents. What do you wish could be different with your parents?"
>
> Teenager: "For one, tell them to stop nagging me all the time, they just don't understand how hard it is for me these days."
>
> Clinician: "So if we could get things better between you and your parents, would that be helpful?" (Clinician seeks out healthy goal of improving the relationship between the teenager and parents.)
>
> Teenager: "Sure, that would make things better."
>
> Clinician: "Any other things you wish could be different?" (Clinician continues to ask about more goals ....)

MIRACLE OF MIRACLES

One of the most popular solution-focused strategies for uncovering the client's goals is called "the miracle question" as described by de Shazer [2]. Although the exact wording will differ depending on the interviewer, the question works by shifting the patient's focus to the future and by tapping into the power of the patient's imagination to envision life without the problems that brought the patient to seek help.

> Clinician: "Imagine that tonight you go to bed, like you normally do. Then, imagine that while you're asleep.... [pause)] ...a miracle happens. Imagine that because of this miracle, your depression [or whatever the patient's problem is] goes away. What will your day be like tomorrow?"
>
> Patient: "Well, I guess I would wake up, and rather than sleep in, I'd wake up on time and get ready instead of procrastinating. Then I'd eat breakfast rather than skipping it, and at breakfast, we'd all get along better without fighting. Then I'd go to work, and I'd have more confidence, so I would say 'no' to people if they ask me to do too much..."

From this brief exchange alone, the clinician would have learned that some possible goals could include (1) helping the patient wake up on time (which may thus involve helping the patient have better sleep hygiene and go to bed on time); (2) eating breakfast; (3) improving relationships at home; and (4) being more assertive at work. These are goals that the patient wants. These are the goals that the patient might readily agree to set.

Thus, if in the initial interview the interviewer and patient jointly agree to work on these goals, the patient will be much more inclined to a positive view of the interviewer. The alliance is off and running. One must never forget that the main goal of the first interview is to make sure that there is a second one. Once the alliance is better established, the clinician may be much more effective subsequently in helping the client address some new goals that may be more important and that perhaps may require more motivation to address, such as character flaws, substance abuse problems, or anger control issues.

MOTIVATIONAL INTERVIEWING: THE ART OF TRANSFORMING UNHEALTHY GOALS AND TASKS

Patients may report unhealthy goals or tasks. Examples include not taking appropriately prescribed medications or harmful behaviors such as substance abuse, self-injury, or suicide.

With topics such as suicide, one of the first obstacles an interviewer must tackle when uncovering the client's goals is a paradoxical one. Interviewers may find that, consciously or unconsciously, they do not want to hear the patient's goals because of the potential ramifications (eg, need for involuntary commitment, need for a prolonged assessment, need for collaborative calls or consultations, or the clinician's own biases about suicide).

To address this obstacle, an innovative and flexible interview strategy has been developed. This strategy–the Chronological Assessment of Suicide Events (the CASE Approach)–was designed to help clinicians uncover suicidal goals and intent effectively and reliably, despite their own hesitancies about asking or the client's hesitancies about sharing [6].

Once problematic client goals have been uncovered successfully, various strategies have been discussed to transform unhealthy, maladaptive, and regressive goals into healthy, progressive, and adaptive ones, such as exploring for the healthy goals that usually lie beneath unhealthy goals and tasks [7].

Getting teenagers to share their unhealthy goals often is quite a challenge because, more often than not, teenagers do not willingly choose to see psychiatrists. They are more like reluctant visitors or even more like the mandated patient. Therefore one cannot necessarily use the strategies that would work with more willing participants.

With such teenagers, and with some adults as well, narrative techniques offer a possible solution. The narrative techniques, described by White and Epston [8], offer a way by which a problem (eg, an unhealthy goal or task) can be externalized outside the person, so that the clinician and client can ally together against the problem. Examples include such questions as "If it were possible, would you like to limit the way that alcohol pushes you around? ... How has alcohol been tricking you into withdrawing and avoiding people? ... What would life be like if alcohol weren't around anymore?"

Of all the approaches to transforming a client's reluctance to change, by far the most influential has been the concept of motivational interviewing first delineated in 1991 by Miller and Rollnick [9] in their classic book, *Motivational Interviewing: Preparing People to Change Addictive Behavior.*

Motivational interviewing was designed originally for substance abuse treatment, which is a classic example of a situation in which forming a therapeutic alliance is challenging because clients prefer their unhealthy goal or task (eg, abusing alcohol or drugs). Motivational enhancement techniques can be helpful when the clinician wants to promote a healthy or positive behavior (eg, seeing a counselor, taking appropriately prescribed medications, smoking or drinking cessation, or adopting healthier lifestyle habits such as eating more healthily).

The following example demonstrates some of the motivational interviewing techniques that can be used to form an alliance when faced with a patient who initially maintains an unhealthy goal. The reluctant client has been brought to the emergency room for suicidal ideation and is being seen by the clinician, who has done some initial history and is now trying to establish a better alliance:

> Clinician: "What would make today's (emergency room) visit helpful?" (Clinician asks for goals.)
>
> Patient: "I want to kill myself, just let me die..." (Patient states unhealthy goal/task.)
>
> Clinician: "I'm sure you must have your reasons for feeling that way... What makes you want to hurt yourself?" (Clinician searches for underlying healthy goal.)
>
> Patient: "I just can't stand the depression anymore; and all the fighting at home. I just can't take it." (The underlying healthy goal/task may be trying to cope with depression and fighting.)
>
> Clinician:"I think I understand—so we need to find a way to help you cope with the depression and the fighting. You told me yourself that there used to be less fighting at home. What would it be like if we found a way to reduce the fighting, have people getting along more?"
>
> Patient: "A lot better, I guess. But it's probably not going to happen."
>
> Clinician: "Okay, I can see why you're frustrated, and I do understand that probably the depression makes it hard to see hope. But I believe that there is a part of you that is stronger and more hopeful, because otherwise you wouldn't be here talking with me." (Clinician externalizes unhealthy thoughts or behaviors as being part of the depression and tries to help the patient ally against the depression.) "That hopeful part of you said that your mood used to be happy. What would it be like if we could get your mood happy again?"
>
> Patient: "A lot better, I guess..."
>
> Clinician:"Just to help me make sure I'm getting this right then, what would you like to see different with your mood?" (The clinician reinforces the client's goals by having the client articulate them.)
>
> Patient: "I want to be happy again."
>
> Clinician: "And at home, what would you like to see with how people get along?"
>
> Patient: "I want us to get along better."
>
> Clinician: "Let's agree then, that we will work together on finding a way to help people get along, as well as help your mood get better. How does that sound?" (Clinician paraphrases patient's healthy goals.)
>
> Patients: "Sounds good... (Patient agrees with goals.)

Even after agreement on goals, clients may have unhealthy tasks. For example, the clinician and client may agree on reducing the depression, but the client may believe that an unhealthy task, such as using marijuana, is the best strategy. One possible avenue in such situations might be to agree to give the client a chance to try his or her strategy but to also agree that, if the strategy does not work, something different needs to be tried.

Additional questions can be used to help the client to

- See alternative tasks (eg, "Are there any other ways to help you cope with stress?")
- See that the task is unhealthy. This process might start by asking about positives of the behavior, to help the client feel validated, followed by asking about negatives of the behavior (eg, "What are the positives about using marijuana?"; "What are the negatives about using marijuana?"; "How does the self-cutting work for you?"; "How does the self-cutting work against you?")

Motivational interviewing, as well as Bordin's [1] transtheoretical stages in forming the therapeutic alliance, bears striking similarities to Prochaska and colleagues [10] transtheoretical stages of change model, another model that is well worth exploring and which is quite popular among clinicians in both substance abuse programs and community mental health work. According to Prochaska and colleagues [10], the main stages of change are

1. Precontemplation: The client has no intention to change and is unaware of a problem. In other words, there is no agreement on goals.
2. Contemplation: The client is aware of a problem and would like to change it but has not yet made a commitment to take action. In other words, there is agreement on goals but not yet agreement on tasks.
3. Preparation: The client intends to take action in the near future. In other words, there is agreement on goals, but agreement on tasks is just beginning.
4. Action: The client is taking action to overcome problems. In other words, there is agreement on goals and task.

THE MEDICATION INTEREST MODEL: THE FINE ART OF COLLABORATIVE INTERVIEWING

Shea [11], in his book *Improving Medication Adherence: How to Talk with Patients About Their Medications,* has delineated a model that integrates the principles discussed in this article into a flexible approach for motivating patients to improve their medication adherence, as well as increasing their initial interest in trying a medication. Shea suggests that much of the alliance that forms between patients and any clinician prescribing medications or involved with medication management (eg, psychiatrists, nurses, and psychiatric case managers) evolves from the dialogue unfolding over the use of the medications.

In essence, the medication interest model suggests that the macrocosm called "the patient/physician alliance" often is a reflection of the microcosm called "prescribing and discussing medications." To a large extent, a patient determines how trustworthy and caring a clinician is, as well as how good a listener he or she is, by how the clinician introduces the idea of medications, listens to the patient's concerns about side effects, and is willing to change medication recommendations flexibly based upon the patient's input. According to the model, even the language used to describe this process should be changed from oppositional terms such as "medication compliance" and "medication adherence" to the much more collaborative term "medication interest."

It is useful to see the medication interest model at work in actual clinical practice. About 40 different interviewing techniques for increasing medication interest have been developed. One is called the "inquiry into lost dreams." This technique was first described by a pediatrician in one of Shea's workshops, who was talking about the difficulties of getting a reluctant teenager to take medications for his asthma, but it is just as useful in motivating patients who have mental illnesses, such as depression, obsessive-compulsive disorder, or bipolar disorder.

This particular interviewing strategy is a nice way to wrap up this article, because it integrates and illustrates many of the points discussed here. By using this strategy the clinician helps the client bring forth his or her own personal goals. At the same time the clinician and the client collaboratively choose a task for achieiving those goals (no easy feat when the client is a leery asthmatic teenager in the room with an adult clinician suggesting side-effect-laden medications).

For many of these adolescents, the key to improving their medication interest lies not so much in their desire for relief from something that the asthma has given them (acute breathing problems) as their desire to regain something that the asthma has taken from them (lost dreams). There is no better way to describe this technique than listening to the pediatrician's own words as recorded in Shea's [11] book:

> I find it useful with my kids with asthma to ask them this question or a variation of it, "Is there anything that your asthma is keeping you from doing that you really wish you could do again?" What I find with this age group is that there is often a quick answer to this question, and the answer is often related to a sport, say, football or soccer.
>
> What I find to be so useful about this question is that it opens the door for adolescents, who by definition are prone to form oppositional relationships with adults, to tell me what they want me to do for them. They are calling the shots, not me. The oppositional field seems to dissolve away. Meanwhile, I gain a deeper insight into their motivation for seeking help from their asthma that goes beyond their desire for symptom relief. I might never have known this powerful motivator had I not asked. I can use this knowledge to enhance the adolescent patient's desire to start a medication and to stay on it.
>
> First, although I never provide false hope, if I feel it is within reason, I can use this newly uncovered information immediately to help shape a shared agenda with a comment like, "Now I can't promise this, but I have had some very good luck with helping other students, with asthma like yours, to get back into sports. We have some great meds that can help with that goal. Once again, no promises, but I would like to work with you to see if we might be able to get you back out on that soccer field. How does that sound to you?"
>
> Second, in the future, if there are tough side effects or if the stigma concerns so often seen with kids having to take meds at school become

problematic, I can say something like, "I know you are getting some tough side effects - and they are tough - but, fortunately, I have some ideas on how we might be able to make them much better, and I don't think we have yet seen the full power of these meds to help you feel better. We are still trying to get you back on that soccer field that we talked about in our first meeting. If you can give me another two weeks to see if I can lower the side effects and get you some better relief from these attacks, I think I might be able to do that. Is it a deal?"

The pediatrician has elegantly accomplished exactly what Bordin [1], the solution-focused therapists, and the motivational interviewers have advised: seek out the goals of the client and get client's input on what tasks the client wants to use to achieve these goals. Even the pediatrician's very last phrase, "Is it a deal?", turns control over the decision to use a new task (making a medication change) over to the teenager. Translated into psychiatric practice, the inquiry into lost dreams question simply becomes, "Is there anything that your OCD [or whatever other psychiatric disorder is the focus of treatment] is keeping you from doing that you really wish you could do again?"

SUMMARY

I hope that you will find this introduction to solution-focused interviewing, motivational interviewing, and the medication interest model to be of immediate value in your clinical practice. I have found that these approaches provide a fresh perspective on the engagement process, a phenomenon that will always provide moments of fascination and, if handled well, will provide patients with moments of healing.

References

[1] Bordin E. The generalizability of the psychoanalytic concept of the working alliance. Psychotherapy: Theory, Research and Practice 1979;16:252–60.

[2] de Shazer S. Clues: investigating solutions in brief therapy. New York: W.W. Norton & Company; 1988.

[3] Budman S, Hoyt M, Friedman S. The first session in brief therapy. New York: The Guilford Press; 1992.

[4] Miller S, Hubble M, Duncan B. Handbook of solution-focused brief therapy. San Francisco (CA): Jossey-Bass; 1996.

[5] de Jong P, Berg I. Interviewing for solutions. New York: Brooke and Cole Publishers; 1998.

[6] Shea SC. The delicate art of eliciting suicidal ideation. Psychiatr Ann 2004;34:385–400.

[7] Book H. How to practice brief psychodynamic psychotherapy. Washington, DC: American Psychological Association Press; 1998.

[8] White M, Epston D. Narrative means to therapeutic ends. New York: Norton; 1990.

[9] Miller W, Rollnick S. Motivational interviewing: preparing people to change addictive behavior. New York: Guilford Press; 1991.

[10] Prochaska J, Norcross J, DiClemente C. Changing for good. New York: William Morrow and Co; 1992.

[11] Shea SC. Improving medication adherence: how to talk with patients about their medications. Philadelphia: Lippincott Williams & Wilkins; 2006.

Practical Interview Strategies for Building an Alliance with the Families of Patients who have Severe Mental Illness

Aaron Murray-Swank, PhD[a,b,*], Lisa B. Dixon, MD, MPH[a,b], Bette Stewart, MS[b]

[a]VA Capitol Network (VISN 5) Mental Illness Research, Education, and Clinical Center (MIRECC), VA Maryland Healthcare System, 6A-157, 10 North Greene Street, Baltimore, MD 21201, USA
[b]Department of Psychiatry, Division of Services Research, University of Maryland School of Medicine, 737 West Lombard Street, 5th Floor, Baltimore, MD 21201, USA

Family members play an integral role in the lives of most persons who have serious mental illness, and the importance of family involvement in the treatment of persons who have serious mental illness is widely recognized. The recent report of the President's New Freedom Commission calls for a care system that is "consumer and family centered" [1]. Moreover, in a large body of randomized trials, family psychoeducation programs have demonstrated robust effects in reducing patient's rates of relapse [2]. Best-practice treatment guidelines of the American Psychiatric Association [3] and other professional organizations strongly recommend family involvement in treatment as a critical element of quality care for persons who have serious mental illness.

This article provides a practical interviewing guide for mental health professionals who work with patients who have serious mental illness and their families. At the outset, we want to emphasize that we write this article as family members of people living with mental illness, in addition to our professional roles as mental health clinicians and researchers who focus on the delivery of services for patients who have a serious mental illnesses (such as schizophrenia, schizoaffective disorder, and bipolar disorder) and their families. This article offers our perspectives grounded in our experience as spouses, siblings, parents, and children of people who have mental illness. By considering this topic from the dual vantage points of both family members and professionals,

*Corresponding author. VA Maryland Healthcare System, MIRECC, 6A-157, 10 North Greene Street, Baltimore, MD 21201. E-mail address: aaron.murray-swank@va.gov (A. Murray-Swank).

0193-953X/07/$ – see front matter
doi:10.1016/j.psc.2007.01.004

we hope to provide a useful roadmap clinicians can use to navigate their work with families.

The article begins by considering the role of the family in the inpatient phase of treatment and then moves to a discussion of working with families while the patient is in outpatient care.

PART I: BUILDING AN ALLIANCE WITH FAMILIES IN INPATIENT SETTINGS

The family experience of mental illness varies substantially, depending on the family member's relationship to the patient (eg, parent, spouse, sibling) and on the patient's diagnosis and phase of illness. There are, however, several typical themes and issues among families who experience the psychiatric decompensation and hospitalization of a loved one.

Common Fears, Anxieties, and Concerns of Family Members

This section addresses three common themes: (1) emotional responses of the family to illness and hospitalization, (2) family expectations of inpatient treatment, and (3) family roles and determining spokespersons.

Emotional responses of the family to illness and hospitalization

As family members, we have experienced the roller coaster of emotional responses that accompany this phase of illness and treatment. Family members often experience profound fear, shock, and trauma related to their relatives' illness and its impact on family life. Their loved one's illness and need for hospitalization is likely to be a time of instability and chaos in the life of the family. Coupled with this tremendous stress, family members may feel a sense of relief when their loved one has "landed somewhere" with their admission to the hospital.

When interviewing family members, clinicians should be attuned to their emotional state and make active efforts to acknowledge and normalize what they might be feeling. Techniques such as reflection (eg, "sounds like you are feeling frustrated") and summarizing statements can help family members feel heard and understood. Another way for a clinician to communicate this message could be

> I realize that you have really been through a lot during this time—you may be feeling anxious, worried, overwhelmed, angry, or maybe a combination of many different feelings—this is certainly understandable, normal, and to be expected as you are dealing with everything going on with [patient's name].

It also is important to realize the impact that family members often feel when visiting their loved one on an inpatient psychiatric unit. One of us can remember the experience of first seeing our loved one hospitalized: "I burst into tears ... it was worse than I could imagine it was."

This initial impact can be particularly jarring to family members who have been involved in an involuntary commitment of their loved one. Confronted with the realities of a locked inpatient unit, the family member can be filled with guilt and second thoughts about having done the right thing. A reassuring comment at the right moment can be greatly comforting:

> Naturally it can be disturbing to see [name] in the hospital. I just want to emphasize that you really did the right thing bringing [name] into the hospital, even though he didn't want to come in. I think you might have saved his life. It took real courage and love to do what you did. And we are going to do everything we can to help him get better. He is very lucky he has you, and that you were there to do what needed to be done to help him.

We have found that it also is useful to be aware of the setting's unique impact on each family member as the family becomes familiar with the unit. For instance, it can be helpful to inquire about family members' experience when first meeting them in the inpatient context. A clinician might say

> Thanks so much for making the time to come in today to meet with me. We believe that your participation in the treatment process is really important. I'm wondering if you have had the opportunity to meet with inpatient staff when [name] has been hospitalized in the past?

It can be helpful to learn what the family's experience has been like in the past to understand how they may be experiencing the current inpatient setting: "I'm also wondering if you have had any particularly good or particularly bad experiences with inpatient staff before?"

This also can be a point at which the clinician can orient the family to the unit and the hospital. Such an orientation and introduction can put family members at ease and also can help the clinician understand "where the family is at" as they are entering the often unfamiliar (and, at times, chaotic and frightening) world of inpatient psychiatric treatment.

Family expectations of inpatient treatment

Families may have a wide variety of expectations of hospitalization and treatment. Particularly in the initial years of illness, family members may have unrealistic expectations that hospitalization will "cure" the problem and return their loved one back to normal upon discharge. It often is frustrating for clinicians to encounter such beliefs, and we certainly have felt these frustrations when working with families in their professional roles. At the same time, it is critical to realize that families' unrealistic expectations typically are not rooted in a willful denial of their loved one's illness. Instead, families' beliefs often reflect a lack of information coupled with an emotional coping process of trying to come to terms with the painful reality of their relatives' illness.

In addressing families' expectations, it can be helpful to provide an orientation to the current context of inpatient care at some point during the family interview. For example, a clinician may explain:

> It is important for you to know what we do here on the inpatient unit and the role that we play in [name's] treatment. Typically, the purpose of

hospitalization is to help get people through a crisis when their symptoms get worse, to provide an environment to ensure their safety, and to make sure they are linked up with outpatient care as they are discharged.

Nowadays, extended periods of hospitalization are pretty unusual for people who have mental illness. Instead, the emphasis is more focused on helping people get back to the community when they are safe and able to return to their living environment. I know this can be difficult for family members, who sometimes experience a sense of relief when their loved ones are hospitalized. It can be frustrating for all of us to deal with the limits of what we can accomplish while [name] is in treatment here.

However, we do hope that we can work with you too, as we help [name] get her illness more under control. We also hope to address your needs for information about [name's] illness and treatment and her plan for care while she is hospitalized here.

This explanation also may serve as a point of entry to discuss sources of support for family members, including professional family services and other education programs and avenues of support for family members. For example, some inpatient units have educational family programs that provide a forum for family members to learn about their loved one's illness. Community resources, such as family education programs offered by the National Alliance for the Mentally Ill, can offer another place to refer families for education and support. As a practical matter, we have found it helpful for staff who interview families to have a current, well-organized repository of information about mental illness and such resources, so information can be provided to families rapidly and smoothly.

Family roles and determining spokespersons
It is important for clinicians who interview families to recognize the ways in which families are organized and the roles that different family members of the patient may play. It is common for one family member to act as the designated spokesperson for the family when the patient is hospitalized. It is critical to take the time to establish a positive bond with this spokesperson, because his or her translations of what the clinician says may be the only information from which the family makes its impression of the care. Also, it is important to realize that the patient's illness often prompts a reshuffling of family roles.

Moreover, as time passes, there may be generational transitions, so that siblings assume a more active role as the patient's parents age. The key point for interviewers is to assess and be sensitive to who in the family are the central figures in the life of the patient. For example, interviewers may ask, "Who is usually involved in helping [name] when he has difficulties?"

Potentially Disruptive Issues for Clinicians in the Inpatient Setting
Contact between clinicians and families may occur in a variety of ways in the inpatient context. Family meetings may be planned during the course of hospitalization. More often, we have found that contact with families happens through a variety of more informal avenues: during family visits to the patient,

family telephone calls to the unit, or telephone calls from the treatment team to the family. This section examines two issues in communication that sometimes can create stress between staff and family: (1) time and (2) confidentiality.

Time limitations

For clinicians, the first difficulty is lack of time. In a common scenario, family members visit and request an unplanned meeting with their loved one's physician or other staff on the unit. Frequently, it is not possible for staff to set aside other duties and make time for such a meeting. In building an alliance with families, however, we believe that it is critical to communicate the message that the clinical team values family input and involvement in treatment. As family members, we have found it frustrating to be "brushed off" by clinical staff completing paperwork or attending to other duties on the unit. Thus, we believe that it is important for staff to be attentive to families, within the context of their limited time and other demands. For example, a busy psychiatrist with only 10 minutes to meet with a visiting family could explain:

> Your input is really valuable, and talking with you is very important to me. I wish I had several hours to review all that we need to talk about. I only have 10 minutes right now, however, so let's set priorities in how we might use our time. Perhaps you could tell me about your main questions and concerns, and we can come up with a plan to make sure you are included in the treatment process while [name] is being treated here.

Confidentiality concerns

Issues of confidentiality can pose particular challenges to clinicians in working with families in the inpatient setting. Professional ethics and organizational policies appropriately require clinicians to obtain the consent of patients before releasing specific information about their treatment to family members (although there can be specific exceptions when safety issues, such as suicide and homicide, are active). This consent typically is documented in a written release-of-information form. Marsh [4] has provided useful guidelines for organizational policy and clinical practice concerning issues of confidentiality, designing appropriate forms, and working with families of patients who have serious mental illness.

Perhaps one of the most difficult and common scenarios is when a family member asks clinicians for information about the patient's treatment, and the patient has not provided permission to release information to family. In such situations, we believe it is important for clinicians first to reinforce the family members' interest in the patient's treatment and in their effort to make contact with the staff. For example: "I am so glad that you called [came in], and that you are interested in learning more about [name's] treatment here."

Next, the clinician should provide a straightforward explanation to the family member regarding the relevant confidentiality issues:

> As you probably know, medical information is private and protected. Therefore, I can't share any specific information about [name's] treatment at this time without her permission. I know it's hard for family members in

> these situations; it is difficult for us, too, because we really value the oppor-
> tunity to include patients' families as part of the treatment whenever we
> can. What I can do is talk with [name] the next chance that I get to try
> to get her permission to talk with you more about her treatment.

It then can be helpful to ask the family members about their needs and offer
information that can be shared, such as answering general questions about psychiatric illness, treatment programs, and resources for family members. For
example:

> I can't share specific information about [name's] treatment, but I would be
> happy to answer more general questions you might have at this time. Do
> you have any general questions about our unit, or about mental illness,
> that I might be able to help with?

Information that can be helpful for families includes a description of the inpatient unit, other treatment resources in the community, programs to support
family members of people who have mental illness, and general information
about psychiatric illness and treatment. Materials also can be sent to family
members to provide this information (eg, brochures or booklets about mental
illness, Internet-based information, flyers about specific programs).

PART II: BUILDING AN ALLIANCE WITH FAMILIES IN OUTPATIENT SETTINGS
Common Fears, Anxieties, and Concerns of Family Members
This section addresses three important themes: (1) unmet needs for informa-
tion/support, (2) differences in opinion on how to help the patient, and (3)
problems in establishing a sound rapport and reliable contact with the treatment team.

Unmet needs for information
Research consistently has documented that family members of people who
have serious mental illness report strong, and often unmet, needs for information and support related to their loved one's psychiatric disorder [5]. In our experience as family members, we have felt the desperation of not knowing where
to find help in coping with the mental illness of a loved one. A lack of knowledge, combined with societal stigma regarding psychiatric disorders, often
leaves family members feeling profoundly isolated in dealing with the many
challenges they face related to their loved one's disorders.

It is important for clinicians to keep in mind that family members may have
varying levels of knowledge about mental illness. Some families may have
a great deal of information about psychiatric disorders, whereas others may
have little knowledge. It is important, therefore, to avoid making assumptions
about family knowledge (or to assume a lack of knowledge). At this point, in
building an alliance with families, we have found it helpful to meet the family
"where they are at" by first supporting the family's desire to be involved and

then asking some introductory questions to assess family members' understanding of their relative's problems. For example:

> Thanks for taking the time to meet with me today about [name's] treatment. To begin, it would be helpful to get your thoughts about the problems that [name] is seeking treatment for. If it is okay with you, I would like to ask you a couple questions to get your input and learn about your understanding of things. Can you tell me a little bit about what you think about [name's] problems?"

Follow-up inquiries can include more focused questions such as:

1. "What do you think has caused [name] to have these problems?"
2. "Has anybody ever given you a diagnosis for his/her problems?" (If they have been told of a diagnosis, it is useful to follow up with a question such as, "What is your understanding of what that diagnosis means?")
3. "Are there things that make things better for [name]?"
4. "Are there things that make things worse?"

Questions such as these can help the interviewer learn about family members' views about their relative's psychiatric problems. In addition, such questions can provide useful information to enhance the patients' treatment. For example, family members often have valuable observations about prodromal symptoms that signal a risk for relapse in the patient. Note that these inquiries avoid using the term "illness," "disorder," or other psychiatric terminology. It is best to avoid using this language and hold off on offering educational information until the interviewer has a good understanding of the family members' view of the patients' problems.

Differences in opinion on how to help the patient

Perhaps one of the most challenging scenarios for the interviewer is when the family has views that are in direct contrast to the current biopsychosocial understanding of psychiatric disorders. For example, family members may believe that the patient just needs to pull him or herself "up by the bootstraps" in dealing with their problems, believing that psychiatric medications are not needed.

In such situations it is helpful to listen attentively and understand the family members' perspectives. To the extent that it is appropriate, it is useful first to validate the family members' concerns or points of view. But the clinician should follow with respectful and culturally appropriate educational information. As in the example given, if a family member opposes medication and believes that the patient just needs to try harder, the clinician can acknowledge this perspective:

> I agree that it's almost always true that people do better if they try harder and if they believe they can be successful. So, it would be really great if Johnny could try harder at cleaning up around the house. But one of the things we are learning about the illness of schizophrenia is that chemical changes in the brain change a person's ability to plan and be organized. It can also reduce a person's ability to feel satisfied and proud of

completing a task. All of these problems limit someone's ability to pull themselves up by the bootstraps.

With regard to medication, an example dialogue may be as follows:

Clinician: "I completely understand your hesitation about medication. Can you help me understand what your concerns are about Johnny taking the medicine?"

Family member: "Well, every time he comes in, it seems like they add more medicines for him to take! And the more medicines you take, the more problems that you get—and I don't see any of them helping."

Clinician: "I'm glad you raise these questions about the medicines he is on, and how they might be affecting him. Let me also say that I know it's frustrating to see such limited progress—I wish we had more effective ways to help people get better quicker. Let's talk more about the role that medications might play in helping Johnny at this time. The overall goal of the medications is to help reduce the symptoms that are part of schizophrenia—things like developing unusual beliefs, not making sense, hearing voices. When Johnny gets sick, these are the kind of symptoms that get worse for him."

Family member: "Yea, he acts pretty crazy sometimes."

Clinician: "For most people, the medicines can help control these kinds of symptoms. They won't make everything better, but controlling these kinds of symptoms is an important first step. You also raised a concern about the number of medicines he is on and the possible side effects of they might have. Let me tell you a little bit about each of his medications, and the possible side effects to watch out for [provides appropriate info on specific medications]. I'm so glad that you raised these questions—things usually work best when we can all work together—Johnny, you, and I—to find the medicines that work best for him and have the fewest negative side effects.

Problems with establishing a sound rapport and reliable contact
with the treatment team

To family members, the array of clinicians who provide mental health services to their loved one—psychiatrists, social workers, nurses, psychologists, vocational counselors, residential staff, case managers—often represent a confusing maze to navigate. In our experience, we have found that it is hard for families to learn the system so as to identify the appropriate contact person for a particular concern. Thus, it can be helpful for interviewers to orient family members to the landscape of services that their loved one is receiving, with a brief explanation of the role that each team member plays and the types of concerns they may be able to address. This type of information helps build an alliance with the family by empowering them to become more knowledgeable allies in the care of their loved one. Family members often benefit from having a "point person" among the array of professionals providing services to their loved one.

A related challenge for families is how to establish contact with different members of the treatment team in the outpatient setting. In building a working alliance with family members in the outpatient setting, it is helpful for interviewers to provide advice about how family members might become involved in care and how they can contact team members. Such advice may vary according to the situation (eg, the patient's willingness to have family involved) and treatment setting. As one example, consider the following example from an interview between a social worker (SW) and the mother (Mrs. Jones) of a patient (Susan). The conversation is focused on how the mother can address her concerns about medications to the patient's psychiatrist:

> Mother: "My main concern is the medicines. You know, Susan seems tired all of the time, like she is totally 'out of it.' "
>
> SW: "Sounds like your main concern is about the medications, and I think you have identified an important issue. I would like to work with you to figure out how to best address these concerns. It seems to me that a good first step might be to talk with Susan's psychiatrist about the medications she is taking. Have you had the opportunity to talk with her doctor who prescribes her psychiatric medicines?"
>
> Mother: "Well, sometimes I drive her to the doctor's appointment at the clinic, but I've never gone in with her to talk to the doctor."
>
> SW: "Let's talk about how you might be able to speak with her doctor. Let me throw out a couple ideas for your to consider—first, you could ask Susan if you could come to one of her appointments and raise your questions about the medicines; another way to approach it might be over the phone."
>
> Mother: "I think it might be easier in person—I would rather sit down and talk with the doctor."
>
> SW: "So, you think coming to one of her appointments might be a good idea—maybe we can go through the steps you can take to get to come to one of her appointments. Have you ever talked with Susan about coming in to meet with her doctor?"
>
> Mother: "No, I've never brought it up. I'm not sure what she would say."
>
> SW: "A good first step might be to talk with Susan about this. I know that she gave me permission to speak with you today, so I think that she will be open to having you meet with the doctor. When you talk with her, it might be good to let her know why you want to come to the appointment—to learn more about her treatment and how to best help her."
>
> Mother: "OK, I can ask her if I can come to the next appointment with her."
>
> SW: "I think that is a great plan. There is one other issue for you to be aware of. As you know, medical information is confidential and protected, and this can be an issue when family members want to talk with professionals. So, if you come into meet with the psychiatrist, Susan would need to give her permission to allow the doctor to speak to you; usually, this involves a written form that Susan would sign. Here is an example of the kind of form that is usually used to do this [shows copy of release-of-information form] …"

In this example, the social worker is actively coaching Mrs. Jones as to how she can get her concerns about the medications addressed with the appropriate member of the treatment team and providing information about potential barriers to family participation (eg, patients' permission, confidentiality issues).

Potential Obstacles for Clinicians in the Outpatient Setting

This section discusses two particularly important problems encountered in the outpatient setting: (1) procuring permission from patients to talk with family members in an ongoing basis, and (2) transforming difficulties encountered while trying to engage family members in ambulatory settings.

Talking with patients about involving family in care

To initiate contact with families, it is necessary to ask the patient to identify members of his or her family and to obtain the patient's permission to speak with them. Although the primary focus of this article is on interviewing family members, these interviews will be brief or nonexistent unless the clinician has done a good job of interesting the patient in involving family members. Consequently, we would like to devote attention to some techniques we have found useful.

Patients have a wide range of family experiences and preferences with regard to family involvement in their mental health care. As an initial starting point, it is important to assess who the patient considers to be their family support system and what role, if any, these individuals may play in helping the patient manage his or her psychiatric disorder. For example one could say, "I would like to ask you some questions to understand your family relationships and support system better. Do you have people you would consider to be your family or are like family to you? Who would those people be for you?"

For many patients, significant "family" and potential allies in treatment may include members of the support network who are not relatives (eg, a friend, pastor, Alcoholics Anonymous or Narcotics Anonymous sponsor). After identifying the key members of the support network, it is helpful to learn about patients' level of contact with these individuals: for example,

1. Does the patient live with a family member?
2. If not, how close do family members live?
3. How often does the patient talk, e-mail, or get together with family members?

Next, it is important to understand the role that these individuals play in supporting the patient, including any involvement in their mental health treatment. For example, one could say, "So, you have said that you are closest to your two brothers, and you get together with them every couple of weeks. I'm wondering if your brothers have been supportive as you have been dealing with your mental illness?"

Patients may have a variety of experiences with family in relation to their illness. Interviewers should use techniques such as summaries and reflections to gain an understanding of the patients' experience and help him or her feel supported. Finally, if it not yet known, the interviewer can assess the degree to which family has been involved in the patient's mental health treatment in the past and the patient's preferences with regard to involving family at this time. For example, one could ask:

1. "Have your brothers been involved in your mental health treatment by coming in to meet with your doctor?"

2. "Have they ever attended any kind of educational programs or groups?"
3. "Would you like to have your brothers involved in your mental health treatment?"
4. "What might be the possible benefits?"
5. "What, if any, are your concerns about having them involved?"

Overall, the goals of this discussion are to help the patient (1) identify family members who could be allies in their treatment; (2) consider the potential advantages of family involvement in treatment; and (3) identify concerns they might have about family participation.

In some instances, the patient may be ambivalent about involving the family. This feeling is understandable, given the complexity of family relationships and the possibility of the presence of abusive family members, as well as the personal nature of mental health treatment. When the patient experiences mixed feelings about involving the family in mental health care, the primary task of the interviewer is to help the patient make informed choices, considering the potential advantages and disadvantages of family involvement in care.

It is particularly important to try to enhance communication with carefully selected family members regarding safety issues such as suicide and violence. Every effort should be made to get permission from the patient to talk openly with key family members (such as a family member or parents with whom a patient is currently living) about these critical issues, for two reasons. First, family members may, in the process of ongoing care, provide life-saving information regarding the patient's risk for suicide and also may be effective partners with the patient and treatment team in suicide prevention plans. Second, it is hard to put into words the stress, fear, and anxiety that family members experience when they are worried that a loved one may attempt suicide. One can imagine the extreme anxiety that a family member can face in making even a simple everyday decision—such as whether to go to work—if there are concerns that leaving the patient alone could result in death by suicide. Family members need guidance from clinicians to navigate these difficult waters effectively. They also can receive great relief—so that they do not fret unduly—from reassurance, when it is appropriate, that "safety concerns are not an issue at this moment."

Good communication, guidance on setting limits, and education on how to react appropriately are also critical for anyone living with a patient who is finding relief through the use of nonlethal self-damaging actions such as self-cutting. By helping family members understand the dynamics of these behaviors and how to respond appropriately without enabling secondary gain, clinicians can provide tremendous relief to the family members and help break the maladaptive cycle of self-cutting itself.

On a final note, never forget that, if suicide is a definite risk, the need to procure the information necessary to perform a sound suicide assessment takes precedence over confidentiality. Information from family members may be life saving in this regard, and at times confidentiality must be broken. If at all possible, in such situations, consult with a supervisor or colleague to decide whether the crisis requires overriding of confidentiality.

Difficulties with engaging family members

Engaging families as allies in the treatment process can be a challenge, particularly in the outpatient setting, in which access to the family can be more limited. It is important to recognize that family members may have reservations about meeting with their loved one's mental health clinicians or participating in family services. For example, family members may be concerned about intruding on their relative's privacy or may be worried that such participation will add additional care-giving demands. Practical barriers, such as limited time, child-care needs, and lack of transportation also may prevent family members from participating in services. Unfortunately, some family members may have past negative experiences with the mental health system or family therapy, given prior outdated theories that emphasized the family environment as a causative influence on mental disorders (eg, the schizophrenogenic mother).

Clinicians should communicate appropriately the message that the illness is not the family's fault and should provide educational information about what is known about the etiology of psychiatric disorders. For example, when given the opportunity, a clinician can explain:

> Relatives often have questions about why their loved one developed schizophrenia. Although the causes are not completely understood, we know that genetics play a big part in determining who is most likely to develop schizophrenia. Also, we know that stressful life events play a role in triggering episodes of the illness. Research has shown that schizophrenia is an illness of the brain. In other words, the symptoms of the illness are caused when certain areas of the brain are not functioning properly, and the chemicals that the brain uses to communicate are out of balance. I want to emphasize that schizophrenia is not caused by parenting or family behaviors. In fact, some of the most loving parents I have ever met have had children who go on to develop schizophrenia. On the other hand, we do know that families can play an important role in helping their loved ones manage and cope with this difficult illness.

To engage families, clinicians must communicate the value of family involvement to both patients and their relatives. Shea [6] describes a variety of interviewing techniques that can help address the underlying fears that family members may bring to the initial meeting. Two of these techniques are particularly germane to this discussion. In the first the clinician openly acknowledges the immense value of the family member's first-hand longitudinal knowledge of both the patient and their care to date:

> One of the things I want to emphasize early on is how important your input and background information are in our helping John. There is no one in the world who knows him better than you. We are dependent on your input. I also really want to know what you think has worked and what you think hasn't.

Shea [6] goes on to describe a common fear of parents that the "new psychiatrist" is going to "screw around with the meds." Many times the patient has been tried on numerous ineffective cocktails of medications, whose painful results have affected both the patient and family members.

Although the urgency of the presenting symptoms may necessitate immediate major medication changes, this situation—in an outpatient setting—is not typical at the time of many first meetings with a family member. With this interviewing technique, the clinician emphasizes that although new medication ideas may be tried—and prove to be quite helpful—nothing is going to be done hastily. Moreover the clinician emphasizes that the ongoing input of the family (if allowed by the patient) will be sought first:

> One of the most foolish things a physician can do is to change the medications before talking with parents and the patient about what is working. Your input is vital. Who knows? We may find some really useful new medications to try, or we may find that his current meds are the best. No matter what, I have no intention of changing anything until I learn more from you on what has and has not worked. By the way, if your son agrees, in the future I would like to talk with you and get your thoughts about any potential major medication changes. At this point in time, what is your opinion about the medications that [patient's name] is taking?''

In their discussion of how to best engage families, Mueser and Glynn [7] offer three useful strategies that interviewers can use to enhance engagement: (1) letting the family know they are not alone; (2) providing support and allowing relatives to vent; and (3) instilling hope for change. In addition to these strategies for interacting with family members, persistence and flexibility are important ingredients in the effort to engage family members as allies in treatment.

For example, clinicians can offer the chance for family members to be involved at multiple points in the treatment process, recognizing the changing needs of the patient and family members. Using individually tailored approaches to invite family members to participate in care (eg, by e-mail, telephone, exchanging written updates) can go a long way toward engaging families successfully.

In summary, in both inpatient and outpatient settings, interviewing families requires a combination of the clinical skills required for working with patients and the communication skills necessary for interacting effectively with colleagues. In many ways, the interviewer is best viewed as a consultant to family members, who often are faced with multiple stresses and challenges and can benefit tremendously from practical information, guidance, and support. By establishing an effective working alliance with patients' families, clinicians enhance the quality of care provided and provide greater opportunities for recovery in their work with persons with serious mental illness.

References

[1] President's New Freedom Commission on Mental Health. Achieving the promise: transforming mental health care in America. SDHHS Publication No. SMA-03-3832, Rockville (MD); 2003.

[2] Murray-Swank AB, Dixon LB. Family psychoeducation as an evidence-based practice. CNS Spectr 2004;9(12):905–12.

[3] American Psychiatric Association practice guidelines for the treatment of schizophrenia. Washington, DC: American Psychiatric Association; 1997.

[4] Marsh D. Serious mental illness and the family: the practitioner's guide. New York: Wiley; 1998.

[5] Tessler R, Gamache G. Family experiences with mental illness. Westport (CT): Auburn House; 2000.

[6] Shea SC. Psychiatric interviewing: the art of understanding. 2nd edition. Philadelphia: W.B. Saunders Company; 1998.

[7] Mueser KT, Glynn SM. Behavioral family therapy for psychiatric disorders. 2nd edition. Oakland: New Harbinger Publications; 1999.

Talking with Patients About Spirituality and Worldview: Practical Interviewing Techniques and Strategies

Allan M. Josephson, MD[a],*, John R. Peteet, MD[b]

[a]Division of Child and Adolescent Psychiatry, Department of Psychiatry and Behavioral Sciences, University of Louisville, 200 East Chestnut Street, Louisville, KY 40292, USA
[b]Department of Psychiatry, Harvard Medical School, 75 Francis Street, Boston, MA 02115, USA

Some things are difficult to talk about with strangers. Religion and spirituality are in that category. The aphorism "don't discuss religion or politics," intended to promote harmonious relations with others, often seems to guide psychiatric interviewing. Until recently, psychiatrists rarely taught trainees to inquire about religion and spirituality, and when they did it was often to investigate its pathologic aspects. Psychiatrists now recognize that these matters are important to much of the populace and that attending to them probably will improve clinical psychiatric practice.

Research increasingly demonstrates that religion and spirituality affect health [1] and mental health in particular [2]. Recognizing the importance of religion and spirituality as a resource, The Accreditation Council on Graduate Medical Education and the guidelines of the Residency Review Committee for Psychiatry now require programs to instruct residents about the religious and spiritual aspects of patients' lives [3]. There is a growing clinical literature on ways in which clinical practice can include consideration of patients' spirituality and worldview [4,5].

Consequently, we felt it was an opportune time to create an article that presents a down-to-earth, practical guide for addressing some of the key interviewing skills needed to explore a patient's framework for meaning—the patient's religion, spirituality, and worldview. The article offers guidelines on the process of the interview, including ways to initiate conversation in this area, with suggestions and specific questions useful for a more thorough exploration of the patient's religious and spiritual life. We have found all these techniques to be useful in our daily practices.

*Corresponding author. E-mail address: allan.josephson@louisville.edu (A.M. Josephson).

0193-953X/07/$ – see front matter
doi:10.1016/j.psc.2007.01.005

Agreement on how best to define religion and spirituality remains elusive, but the authors offer these operational definitions. Spirituality is concerned with the transcendent and the individual's connection to a larger reality or context of meaning. Religion is the form that spirituality takes within given traditions, with basic tenets or beliefs often set within a historical context. The increasingly common term "worldview" is even broader in scope: it refers to a person's philosophy of life [6]. Certainly religious individuals have a worldview, but the use of the term "worldview" allows the inclusion of those who have a set of precepts by which they live and organize their lives even if they do not ascribe to a formal creed or religion.

Clinicians should keep in mind that sometimes a patient's worldview—what makes him or her tick—is rooted firmly not in a spiritual tradition or religious belief but in secular frameworks for meaning such as patriotism, family loyalties, community service, recovery groups (such as Alcoholics Anonymous or Narcotics Anonymous), or the values of a street gang. These frameworks for meaning, which often have a profound impact on daily behavior, are equally important to explore when eliciting a patient' worldview.

GENERAL INTERVIEWING CONSIDERATIONS
The Importance of Spiritual Inquiry

Why is it important to inquire about the spiritual aspect of patients' lives? The rationale for acquiring this information has been elaborated fully elsewhere [7,8]. Simply put, inquiry in this area has the potential to enhance how much we can help people and improve our treatment planning. The term "biopsychosociospiritual" reflects the fact that spirituality may, along with biologic, psychologic, and social factors, impact a variety of issues related to clinical care including contributing to the risk of developing clinical disorders and serving as a protective factor [9]. It also should be noted that religious and spiritual factors may exacerbate or ameliorate a condition that arises from independent sources.

The other benefits of uncovering a patient's worldview include:

1. Religious and spiritual questioning during an interview can improve a treatment alliance, because patients feel that important aspects of their existence are understood.
2. At times patients present religious reasons for resisting treatment recommendations, whether they be pharmacotherapy, psychotherapy, or a specific medical therapy.
3. An understanding of the patient's worldview may be a critical component in a suicide assessment, because a strong belief in a hereafter, in which one can reunite with loved ones, may provide a powerful pull toward suicide if the patient believes that his or her god would forgive the act.
4. An understanding of the moral codes and values by which children are raised—or the effects of the absence of such codes—may have a major impact on the choice of treatment interventions and the client's interest in pursuing them.

A more thorough understanding of the patient's spirituality and spiritual practices can enhance treatment planning significantly. In this regard, Shea

[10] has shown, in a book written to be read by patients, how the interaction of the wings of the biopsychosociospiritual model, an interaction he calls "the human matrix," can be useful in developing a common language for collaborative treatment planning. In matrix treatment planning, the patient's worldview is seen as interacting with intrapersonal factors, biologic and psychologic factors, and the patient's social context. For example, could an intervention consistent with the patient's spirituality (eg, meditation or listening to Gregorian chant) have a positive impact on the patient's biology, perhaps accentuating or replacing the use of an antianxiety agent? Worldview, as an integral aspect of such matrix treatment planning, can help the client and the clinician jointly brainstorm untapped, and often overlooked, avenues for intervention.

The Potential Impact of the Interviewer's Own Beliefs on the Inquiry

The goal of this article is to help contemporary clinicians demystify exploration of the religious and spiritual aspects of their patients' lives, just as a previous generation of clinicians learned to demystify in-depth exploration of a patient's sexual functioning.

Why is this exploration difficult? Griffith and Griffith [11], when exploring this topic in their remarkably thorough and practical book, *Engaging the Sacred in Psychotherapy: How to Talk with People About Their Spiritual Lives*, noted that many therapists reported struggling with how to bring up spirituality. Clinicians often ask: "Why doesn't this topic come up more in my therapies?" and "What are the questions I need to ask?"

In the initial diagnostic interview, subtle references by patients to matters of faith or worldview may not be noticed by some clinicians, may seem an irritating detour to others, and may present inviting opportunities to still others. We view these discrepancies as being powerfully influenced by the clinician's own spiritual beliefs and possible countertransference issues. In addition to clinicians' potential lack of training in exploring spiritual issues, it is likely that their worldview or spiritual position influences what material is followed up and how it is explored. Asking questions about spirituality and worldview implicitly forces the clinician to examine his or her own spiritual life.

Some therapists who have not resolved these questions for themselves may find it disconcerting to ask questions such as "Do you believe in God?", "What are you living for?", or "Do you believe you have a connection beyond the material world?" In part, the therapists' ambivalence may explain why this area might be so difficult to pursue.

Moreover, an interviewer may be hesitant to inquire about a patient's belief in God, because the interviewer fears the possibility of the patient's responding, "How about you, do you believe in God?" Once interviewers have thought through a range of reasonable responses to such a question, they may feel significantly more comfortable inquiring about spirituality during initial assessments and in subsequent therapy.

In the process of interviewing regarding spirituality, a clinician also may need to consider "Why am I having such a strong reaction to this patient?"; "Is my own skepticism about some of these matters an impediment to the therapeutic process?"; "Is my personal interest in this area leading me to focus too much on it?" A careful examination of one's own worldview therefore is essential preparatory work to conducting interviewing that is as unbiased as possible. Our experience, both personally and with our supervisees, is that although even seasoned clinicians practice as if their worldview does not influence the clinical encounter, it undeniably does.

In clinical practice, the clinician either holds the same worldview as the patient or does not. Discrepancies in worldview between the interviewer and the patient can lead to misunderstanding and prejudice in the same way that ethnic and cultural differences can. In such circumstances, it is essential to explore the patient's worldview with an open attitude and unconditional positive regard, always being attuned to indications that the patient rejects the interviewer's worldview perspective.

Sometimes a patient becomes aware that the clinician holds the same worldview as the patient. This knowledge may facilitate the patient's comfort in communicating personal religious beliefs, because the patient realizes that these beliefs will be received without distortion or misunderstanding. At the same time, a similarity in religious background or beliefs can be a liability in the therapeutic relationship and the clinical interview. It may lead to the avoidance of troubling questions that threaten tenets of the faith shared by the client and clinician. A shared similarity in background also may interfere with the clinician's empathy for the patient and preclude an accurate interpretation of the patient's conflicts if the clinician's own faith experience is conflicted [12].

The Risks and Benefits of Self-Disclosure

In most instances there is no need to communicate our worldview to the patient. In some instances, it is clearly inappropriate to do so (eg, when a patient is psychotic or manic). Increasingly, however, therapists are examining whether self-disclosure could occur in some situations. This question is receiving careful attention from the psychotherapeutic community, and the reader is referred elsewhere for a more extensive discussion [13].

Given the potential for inappropriate influence on a patient, the clinician should have a specific clinical reason for volunteering his or her spiritual beliefs, such as when doing so is thought to be necessary to engage the client. Such sharing must be solely for the clinical benefit of the client and never for the personal agenda of the clinician [14]. If such communication takes place, it does so with a clearer rationale when it follows a patient's inquiry rather than being part of a therapist-initiated disclosure.

The following vignette illustrates some of the problems that can arise if a clinician inappropriately communicates his or her worldview and uses that communication to influence the patient:

> A 26-year-old Asian American social worker presented after a hospitalization for a suicide attempt. The psychiatric consultant elicited a history that work stressors following graduation from high school had compounded

lifelong feelings of inferiority. Shortly before becoming suicidal he began seeing an Asian American therapist who, like himself, attended church regularly. The patient reported that the therapy had not been going well because the therapist talked with him about her own religious experiences and her belief that if he committed suicide he would go to hell.

There are, however, situations in which some disclosure serves as a catalyst for therapeutic change and enhances the treatment alliance:

A 19-year-old college student was referred for psychotherapy after a medical evaluation for headaches and abdominal pain revealed no known physical cause. Therapy addressed increasing her self-efficacy and expression of negative affect. She had been subservient to others her entire life, which angered her. In particular, she raged about an authoritarian priest who had insisted that "all anger was sinful and not of God." When the therapist commented, "As I understand the Bible, there were some angry people in there who were quite righteous and good," the young woman visibly relaxed. She responded, "You seem to know my world," to which the therapist continued, "I am not Catholic but I understand something of the life of faith."

Deciding to share one's worldview for clinical reasons, such as engagement of the patient, requires careful attention to boundary issues and presents ethical challenges for the clinician [15]. The clinician always should keep in mind that it is unethical for the clinician to proselytize or to influence a patient's worldview unduly [16]. Effective interviewing gathers the facts necessary to develop a picture of the whole person. Concerns about boundary issues, however well founded, should not prevent exploration of the patient's spirituality. Indeed, we believe that ignoring the worldview of the client—a significant component in the assessment of the whole patient—would raise additional ethical issues [17]. The questions, "What makes this person tick?" and "What are the most important things in her life?" are spiritual questions. Patients often are motivated to discuss what is meaningful to them if asked in sensitive ways.

For many years, it was common for the religiously devout to feel that this area of life would be viewed skeptically by a psychiatrist. For practical reasons alone, clinicians need to take care to be open about spirituality and to suspend judgment and cynicism regarding any faith or spiritual position. When the patient's integrity and personhood are accepted, she probably will feel comfortable in telling her story.

RAISING THE TOPICS OF GOD, RELIGION, AND SPIRITUAL BELIEF
Indirect Methods for Raising Spirituality
Griffith and Griffith [11] offer three practical tips for raising the topic of spirituality in an indirect fashion. First, follow up the patient's own use of religious or spiritually laden language. For instance if the patient uses a phrase such as "By the grace of God I passed the final examination," you might ask something like, "It sounds like God plays a role in your life, is that true?" Second, pursue shifts in emotions that occur related to spiritual themes. Third, facilitate the

interview by appealing to stories of a tradition that a clinician and patient may share.

Griffith and Griffith [11] also have found that indirect questions, such as the following, often lead to fascinating and important self-revelations from clients about their worldviews:

1. For what are you deeply grateful?
2. From where do you draw your strength?
3. Where do you find peace?
4. Who truly understands your situation?
5. When you are afraid or in pain, how do you find comfort?

Such questions may unlock information about important people who may provide rich resources for support. They also make it easy for the client spontaneously to describe spiritual supports such as a personal god or goddess and/or religious beliefs. It is quite informative to see which path the patient chooses.

Additional indirect opportunities to explore worldview occur when patients spontaneously offer that they regularly attend religious services or comment on their life goals. Clothes and jewelry that patients wear (eg, a cross pendant) and objects they bring into the consulting room (eg, books) often are clues to a religious and or spiritual position. Simply pursuing a statement emblazoned on a tee shirt can be productive:

> A 13-year-old boy presented for evaluation of depressive symptoms. He had few vegetative signs of depression, but the interviewer noted a sense of hopelessness and cynicism. The interview was progressing poorly until the clinician noted the boy's tee shirt declaring, "Never underestimate the power of stupid people in large groups." Exploring existential themes of unfairness in life and peer rejection was productive.

There are times when the clinician should note but not pursue religious or spiritual material (eg, when there is strong patient resistance to doing so, or when it has little apparent relevance to the clinical problem). Of course, evidence of conflict in this area may be a reason to explore it further, at least briefly.

> A 45-year-old divorced writer with recently diagnosed colon cancer presented with anxiety about her illness and anger about working with her oncologist, whom she perceived as controlling. When asked in the initial interview if she had been a spiritual or religious person, she emphatically answered "no." Asked to explain, she said she had grown up in a "religious cult" led by her parents, who "practically disowned" her when she left. Her distrust of authority figures based on this early religious experience had stimulated considerable anxiety about depending on a physician with an authoritarian style. In this case, it was fruitful for the clinician to probe gently an apparent end to a line of questioning. On the other hand, although her traumatic religious background helped explain her current symptoms, more detailed questioning may have seemed intrusive.

Direct Methods for Raising the Topic of Spirituality

Most psychiatric interviews are performed with individuals who are obviously symptomatic, reporting and requesting help with problematic thoughts, behaviors, and/or feelings. Although some of these patients also may present with spiritual crises, the majority do not, so the question arises: are there direct methods of raising the topic of spirituality with these individuals who are not coming in spiritual crisis and for whom any talk of spirituality must occur naturally in the context of the disorder being evaluated? Koenig and Pritchett [18] have described a routine screening interview tool (similar to those used to assess vegetative symptoms of depression or a brief marital history) that has become known by the acronym "FICA":

1. (F) Is religious faith an important, daily part of your life?
2. (I) How has this faith influenced your life?
3. (C) Are you currently part of a religious community?
4. (A) Are there spiritual aspects that you would like to address in the development of a treatment plan?

Although these screening questions may elicit responses of limited interest, they often point to areas worth deeper inquiry.

> Jennifer was a 17-year-old high school senior referred for treatment of depression and anxiety, after a negative, extensive workup of physical symptomatology. For the 6 months before referral she had been home schooled, the result of the negative school experience in which she felt ostracized by her peers.
>
> Clinician: How long have you been home schooled?
> Jennifer: Just this year.
> Clinician: How was this decision made?
> Jennifer: I have always attended parochial schools and it has usually worked out. This time, in high school, the group is becoming a clique. My parents said I should stop going there.
> Clinician: Parochial school? Is your family a family of faith?
> Jennifer: Faith! Faith! That's my whole problem.
> Clinician: You really have strong feelings associated with your faith. Tell me about your experience.

In this instance, a simple, even self-evident request to elaborate on her educational experience led to an angry, emotional response. In asking about the word "parochial," the clinician opened up a discussion of significant religious conflicts. Further interviews demonstrated that these conflicts were related directly to her symptoms.

Here are three other direct questions that can provide graceful methods for raising the topic of worldview. The first one, in particular, makes sure that the patient has a chance to describe any of the nonreligious worldviews mentioned earlier in the introduction to this article:

1. People vary in what makes them tick. For some it is religion, for others it is their family, for others it is their community, and, of course, it could

be a combination of things. What would you say makes you tick?

2. People vary in their spiritual beliefs from believing in a god to being agnostic to being an atheist. How would you describe your own beliefs?

3. When you were a child did your parents raise you with a specific religious belief?

GOING DEEPER

A number of situations, not all as dramatic as the one seen with Jennifer, call for a more in-depth exploration. We will consider two areas in particular.

Moral Concerns

Most humans are defensive about moral failings, and there may be no area more difficult to explore. Moral choices and failures, however, can be related to dysphoric states, if not disorders. Sheehan and Kroll [19], in a survey of psychiatric inpatients, found that a substantial minority of patients believed moral transgressions played some role in the development of their illnesses. The majority was not psychotic. Sheehan and Kroll wrote, "Most physicians provide their patients with a biological reductionistic explanation as to the etiological mechanisms of disease and assuredly gloss over the moral or transcendental import of the disease to the ill person."

Clinicians may be able to explore moral concerns more deeply at clinically appropriate points, by asking, for example: "Do you feel your problems developed as the result of making a morally wrong decision?" or "Are you having trouble deciding what is the right thing to do?" or "Are you having trouble forgiving yourself (or someone else)?" Affirmative answers to these questions lead directly to spiritual questions about the process of forgiveness [20].

At times, the intersection of morality and clinical issues can be dramatic:

A 52-year-old woman finally was apprehended for her role as an accomplice in a murder many years earlier. She described relief at shedding her assumed identity, and she related that guilt, anxiety, and depression had plagued her for years as she harbored the knowledge of her wrongdoing. She described several trials of antidepressant therapy as well as psychotherapy that had been unsuccessful. Her arrest and legal accountability resulted in the relief of her symptoms [9].

Existential Issues

Existential crises associated with feelings of meaninglessness, despair, and helplessness, occasioned by medical illnesses or serious disruptions in interpersonal relationships or religious beliefs (eg, feeling abandoned by God), can mimic depression and even lead to suicide. Such crises require interviewing with an existential focus. Questions designed to identify existential themes as well as spiritual resources include: "Where do you find the strength to cope?"; "What means most to you at this point in your life?"; "What are you are living for?"; "Where do you find love and peace?"; and, with terminally ill patients, "How do you feel about the approach of death?"

> A 64-year-old lawyer described his lack of energy and general hopelessness by commenting, "I am not very optimistic about people." After this clue, not specifically religious or spiritual but suggesting existential angst, the therapist merely asked, "Could you tell me more?" At this question, the patient launched into a long description of his view that "people, given the opportunity, will always choose evil over good," that "moral codes barely keep people under control," and that "at the end of the day, evil and darkness will surface in most people." Finally he stated, "The world will do you in if you are not careful." Here a simple, encouraging question revealed hopelessness and a despairing worldview.

Raising children presents existential challenges, leading to moral conflict over spiritually based values if parents' goals for their children differ.

> A successful businessman was contemplating a significant job offer, just as his 16-year-old daughter was recovering from anorexia nervosa. When challenged by a clinician about the advisability of moving when his daughter remained vulnerable to relapse, he stated, "Sometimes you need to climb the mountain." A bitter argument with his wife ensued, ending with her rhetorical question, "What's important in life, anyway?" [9].

RISK AND PROTECTIVE FACTORS

In formulating a case, the mental health clinician will want to consider whether the patient's religion and spirituality is constructive (an integrating resource), destructive (contributing to psychopathology), or both:

1. Religion and spirituality can provide a flexible structure that encourages self-control and a discipline that respects the rights of others. This benefit is particularly true in the areas of aggression and sexuality, where moral codes protect human relationships from being exploitative. Religion and spirituality can be pathogenic when the rules they reinforce become rigid, unyielding, and regarded as ends in themselves.
2. Religion and spirituality can affirm relationships. The sacred religious writings and the modeling of religious leaders typically affirm the rights of others and the inestimable value of persons. Betrayal by religious or spiritual leaders can be traumatic and destructive of a patient's ability to trust.
3. A spiritual worldview may affirm relationships and strengthen basic trust in other individuals and humanity at large, facilitating supportive relationships within families. On the other hand, religious parents can be destructive if, in trying to protect their children from an evil world, they stunt the development of healthy adaptive capacities.
4. Religion and spirituality often provide an intellectual framework by which to manage existential anxiety and doubt. The concept that life has meaning and purpose seems to buffer many stressful situations. Distorted religious beliefs, however, can be damaging to mental health when they preclude the use of medication or assert that the devout do not get depressed.
5. Spiritual and religious communities often provide individuals with support, social relationships, and personal identity which can buffer life stresses,

decreasing the risk of psychiatric disorders. Conversely, the expectations of a religious community can be burdensome to an individual who desires to live outside the community's norms.

Keeping these general risk and protective factors in mind will assist the interviewer in gathering more detailed information about whether the patient's spirituality is a resource or a detriment. This information is supplemented further by the clinician's specific line of inquiry informed by developments in psychiatric epidemiology. For example, most clinicians inquire about a history of abuse in patients who have borderline personality disorder because this association has emerged from the literature. The psychiatric literature is developing quickly in the area of the epidemiology of spirituality and religion, suggesting specific questions regarding spirituality that could be asked when assessing disorders such as depression, substance abuse, and anxiety disorders.

Kendler and colleagues [21] noted in a large twin study that religious devotion buffered the effects of stress in depression-prone individuals. Koenig and colleagues [1] have noted that studies of adolescents and young adults consistently demonstrate an inverse relationship between substance abuse and religious involvement. Sexual problems also require questioning regarding spirituality and worldview. Weaver and colleagues [22] noted that religious involvement of the family and a teenager's religious commitments play an important role in delaying the onset of sexual intercourse. This finding has increasing clinical relevance because recent data suggest an increased incidence of depression with premature sexual activity in young girls [23].

On the other hand, some negative associations are emerging also. One study noted that when church-going youth were sexually active, they were less likely to use contraceptives than non–church attendees [24]. This article cannot review fully the associations between disorders and the risk and protective factors offered by religion and spirituality. It is important, however, for any clinician to be aware of this developing science and its database, which can help inform any rational interview process.

Systematic interviewing in the following areas can complete a spiritual and religious inventory and, in combination with previous explorations, provide a more in-depth understanding of the patient's spiritual problems and resources. Although touched upon in the initial interview, in-depth explorations, such as the following, usually are done during ongoing therapy.

SIX AREAS FOR IN-DEPTH EXPLORATION
Development: What Were You Taught?
Families are the first place an individual receives spiritual instruction (or lack thereof), and interviewing about spiritual development fits naturally into a general review of the patient's experience in her family of origin. Many individuals remain within their family's tradition; others rebel or change spiritual perspective, some through a "conversion experience." These transitions often occur at times of stress and can have profound effects on future development. Such a conversion

should be explored fully, reviewing antecedents, accompanying events, and subsequent behavioral integration of the change in spiritual perspective.

Developmental experience often is conveyed by metaphor as a way of conceiving one thing in terms of another. The patient may describe the constancy of faith positively ("My faith was an island in a sea of trouble") or painfully relate an upbringing that was "a living hell." Such comparisons are a potentially rich area for clinical exploration. When a patient says, "I'm a recovering Catholic," comparing her faith to illness or addiction, a clinician could respond simply by asking, "What are you recovering from?" The interviewer also could stay with the metaphor by asking, "Did certain treatments help you recover from this condition?" Or the interviewer could offer his or her own metaphor, such as, "As I hear you describe your spiritual background, it seems it was a ball and chain, holding you back."

Specific questions with which to explore development might include:

- Did you attend religious services or receive spiritual instruction growing up?
- Was there a spiritual emphasis in your family?
- What was your family's religious tradition? And how did they practice that tradition?
- Was religion a source of conflict between your parents?
- What experiences helped shape your beliefs?
- Did your parents behave in a manner consistent with their beliefs?
- Are your beliefs similar to, or different from, those of your parents?
- Growing up, were other people important to you in your spiritual development?

Community: Where Do You Belong?

Belonging to a spiritual or religious community can be a source of support for those suffering from psychiatric problems, but conflicts within the community or the expectations of the community also can be a source of stress [25]. Community is about belonging, a value of enduring importance and one that may be harder to find in contemporary society. A religious community typically is more organized, often requiring formal membership, whereas a spiritual community is a broader, more loosely knit network. Consider the meaning of community for Ms. AB, recently bereaved of her grandmother:

Dr. X: It sounds like your grandma's funeral was meaningful.

Ms. AB: I got to share memories of grandma with all the other people there who loved her, and I got to be with her one last time in a place that she loved and where we had spent so much time together.

Dr. X: The church?

Ms. AB: That's right.

Dr. X: What did it mean to you that her funeral was in the church?

Ms. AB: I hadn't thought about it, really, because I think all funerals ought to be in a church. But I guess it is the fact that the church represents God, and it's God who creates us and is there at our very beginning and the end, no matter what happens in between. And it's where all the people who have known you the best and longest are.

Ms. AB shows what Allport and Ross [26] would have described as intrinsic religiosity. Her participation in a religious community reflected her deeply internalized beliefs and values. By contrast, individuals with extrinsic faith are those who take part in community purely for social reasons. Specific questions about a patient's religious or spiritual community could include:

- What is your community? To whom do you belong?
- What does your community expect of you?
- What does it do for you?
- Do the leaders of the community communicate with clinicians? How? [11]

Beliefs: What Is Your World View?

Because, as cognitive therapists point out, the "thought is the mother to the deed," an examination of the patient's beliefs elucidates not only how individuals make sense of the world but how they are inclined to act. For example, the common if implicit religious belief that an aspect of the person (a "soul") lasts forever contrasts with the atheist's belief that humans are passing products of time and chance.

Interviewing should assess the clinical impact of a deeply held belief and not merely its presence. For example, the conservative Christian belief that the world is a "sinful, fallen place" is clinically relevant if it causes parents to prevent their children from engaging in developmentally appropriate experiences.

Statements of belief in propositional truth and theological dictates that may be more rigidly required for one to be considered a genuine member of a specific religion can engender conflict. Spirituality itself rarely takes the form of propositional statements and can seem safer to discuss than religion. More rigid religious beliefs often deserve inquiry, however; defensiveness about them can indicate their importance and justify sensitive, respectful exploration. In addition, the personal interpretation that a patient gives to religious stories can provide important clues to the patient's psychologic functioning [9,11].

It is important to ask about both broader theological beliefs and the implications of those beliefs for daily living and personal conduct. Clinicians now have a number of resources available for educating themselves about positions on life taken by the major traditions [4,27]. Are the patient's beliefs convictions or assumptions? Are they conservative or liberal?

Interviewing about core beliefs also should include attention to timing. In most cases, in-depth interviewing in this area should occur only after a therapeutic relationship has been established. Discussion about beliefs can turn quickly into a negative experience for patients, particularly in interviews conducted by inexperienced clinicians who may miss subtle cues about what material to pursue and what to leave unexplored. Some questions about beliefs could include:

- What would you describe as your single most important belief?
- How do you determine what is right and wrong?
- How do you believe most other people determine what is right and wrong?

- Do you have religious and spiritual beliefs that cause you conflict? Do you believe in an after life?
- How do you believe marriage and child rearing should be structured?
- What is success?
- What is the good life?
- What is happiness?
- Do you believe in absolute values?

God: Is There an Ultimate Source of Life?

One foundational question about belief deserves special attention: "Do you believe in the existence of God?" The answer to this question divides individuals into those who believe there is ultimate purpose in life and those who believe that life is the product of time and chance. Interviewing about religion and spirituality flows from this basic categorization.

Asking about a person's perception of what God is like also is informative because one's mental representation of God is intimately connected to one's perceptions of parents or other important authority figures in life [28]. Asking a patient to elaborate on his or her image of God helps the clinician understand the patient's internalized object relations.

Further, a clinician will want to know what role belief in God plays in the patient's life. Freud [29] hypothesized that belief in God was a way of dealing with feelings of helplessness and wishes for parental protection. Although this global statement has been largely discredited, it is not totally without merit. The clinician must consider both hypotheses. Does the patient's belief in God serve an integrating, maturing function by helping the patient function independently and responsibly? Or, in recognizing that he or she is not self-made and owes his or her existence and allegiance to a higher authority, does it seem to justify dependence and avoidance of responsibility (eg, "God must have wanted me to do that.")?

Questions to ask after "Do you believe in God"? include:

- What led you to this belief?
- If you do not believe in God, what led you to this unbelief?
- What are God's most meaningful characteristics?
- How does God affect your personal experience?
- Does your belief in God support coping with problems?

Rituals and Spiritual Practices: How Do You Conduct Your Life?

Rituals as symbolic behavioral expressions of belief allow social participation in celebrations of historical events important to a particular faith tradition. As in the case of the funeral for Ms. AB's grandmother, experiences of awe and wonder are more powerful when shared with others of like belief.

Although the terms "ritual" and "ceremony" often are used synonymously, some distinguish ceremony as a prescribed social behavior, choreographed to proclaim order in the face of life's uncertainties (eg, a graduation ceremony), from ritual as an encounter with the numinous world [11]. For example, rituals such as prayer, meditation, and religious songs stir emotions of wonder and reverence, whereas ceremonies such as inaugurations tend to reinforce certainty and conviction. In reality, ritual and ceremony often merge. For example, religious rituals that evoke awe and wonder, such as Sabbath in the Jewish week and Ramadan in the Muslim calendar, may be repeated to become regular ceremonies.

What function does a given ritual serve in the patient's life? Is it a maladaptive, obsessional means of binding anxiety and fear or an occasion for joy, whether religious (eg, Easter) or developmental (eg, birthdays; anniversaries) that functions to foster peace and the integration of one's relationships with others? Rituals driven by psychopathology are associated with urgency or compulsion rather than with choice, ease, and anticipation. Adaptive rituals are associated with values and beliefs that have significant meaning for the individual in contrast to irrationally held beliefs that cause distress.

> Dr. X: And what gave you peace after your grandmother died?
> Ms. AB: Just knowing that grandma had all her friends around her and she was at peace with God. I'll never forget her funeral. She had all her favorite hymns and Bible passages picked out, and she planned her funeral to be what she called a "Good-bye World, Hello Heaven Party." For a funeral, it really was a great day—the only thing missing was grandma! And the words of the service itself were so comforting, like my grandma herself was there hearing the same words that she heard at funerals when she was a child, and the same words and songs that will be at my funeral and millions of other people's funerals. The same words, and songs, and rituals that connect the dead with the living with those already in heaven, no matter who they were on earth. That made me feel like I was going to be OK without her here in person, because lots of what she loved is staying with me.

Rituals often mitigate the social differences of wealth, social status, race, culture, and power. C.S. Lewis, the brilliant scholar and lay theologian, was asked why he attended church when he was unlikely to learn anything new there. He replied that singing hymns and offering prayers beside uneducated laymen was a powerful ritual for him, reinforcing that all humankind is the same before God.

Questions that can help the clinician distinguish between healthy rituals and those of psychopathological origin include:

- What does prayer mean to you? How and how often do you pray?
- Do you pray alone or with others?
- How often do you engage in meditation or private religious practices that include the study of scriptures?
- How often do you attend spiritual or religious services?

Spiritual Experiences: Do You Have Experiences Beyond Words?

Spiritual experiences transcend the patient's material, day-to-day life. They are linked closely with ritual and ceremony and are components of these events but tend to be individual and not necessarily shared with others. They may be linked to beliefs but can occur apart from explanatory constructs, later taking on meaning within the patient's narrative (eg, as life-changing out-of- body or conversion experiences).

Patients typically find it difficult to put these experiences into words because they defy explanation. A specific type of spiritual experience—the mystical experience—is, by its very definition, beyond words and has been reported across essentially all religions. It typically is marked by intense feelings of a oneness with the godhead, in which a sense of personal self dissolves, time seems to disappear, and one feels an indescribable certainty of the importance of the eternal Now, as well as an almost overpowering sense of compassion. Spiritual experiences, such as those seen in mystical revelations, often involve an intense awareness of physiologic states (as seen in meditative practices); behaviors such as fasting can heighten this awareness further.

Just as psychiatry has been reluctant to incorporate an awareness of the patient's worldview and belief system, it similarly has paid relatively little attention to understanding spiritual experience. Consider the following questions as a guide to interviewing in this area:

- Have you had experiences that you or others would describe as spiritual?
- Have you told others about your experiences?
- How important is spiritual experience in your life?
- Have spiritual experiences led to behavioral changes in your life?
- Does your sense of the presence of a higher power change how you approach personal decisions?
- Do you think you have ever had a mystical experience?

SUMMARY

Asking about a patient's worldview and spiritual concerns in the initial diagnostic interview is a daunting task but is worth the effort. Getting to the heart of the patient's concerns improves patient care and deepens the clinician's understanding of the patient. At the very least, asking the larger questions of life lessens the chance that the patient's experience of the interview will mirror that of a despondent physician who had just been interviewed by a psychiatrist [30]:

I don't think he heard me . . . Depression may be the disease, but it is not the problem. The problem is my life. . . .. It's falling apart. My marriage. My relationship with my kids. My confidence in my research. My sense of purpose. My dreams. Is this depression? . . . I want this depression treated, all right. There is something more I want, however. I want to tell this story, my story. I want someone trained to hear me. I thought that was what psychiatrists did.

References
[1] Koenig HG, McCullough ME, Larson DB. Handbook of religion and health. New York: Oxford University Press; 2001.

[2] Koenig HG, editor. Handbook of religion and mental health. San Diego (CA): Academic Press; 1988.

[3] American Medical Association. Program requirements for residency education in psychiatry. In: Graduate Medical Education Directory, 2002–2003. Chicago: American Medical Association; 2002. p. 309–17.

[4] Josephson A, Peteet J, editors. Handbook of spirituality and worldview in clinical practice. Washington, DC: American Psychiatric Publishing, Inc; 2004.

[5] Josephson A, Dell ML. Religion and spirituality. Child Adolesc Psychiatr Clin N Am 2004;13(1):xv–xvii and 1–230.

[6] Nicholi AM. Definition and significance of a worldview. In: Josephson AM, Peteet JR, Josephson A, et al, editors. Handbook of spirituality and worldview in clinical practice. Washington, DC: American Psychiatric Publishing, Inc; 2004. p. 3–12.

[7] Josephson A, Wiesner I. Worldview in psychiatric assessment. In: Josephson A, Peteet J, editors. Handbook of spirituality and worldview in clinical practice. Washington, DC: American Psychiatric Publishing, Inc; 2004. p. 15–30.

[8] Richards PS, Bergin AE. A spiritual strategy for counseling and psychotherapy. Washington, DC: American Psychological Association; 1997. p. 171–99.

[9] Josephson A, Peteet J. Worldview in diagnosis and case formulation. In: Josephson A, Peteet J, editors. Handbook of spirituality and worldview in clinical practice. Washington, DC: American Psychiatric Publishing, Inc; 2004. p. 31–46.

[10] Shea SC. Happiness is: unexpected answers to practical questions in curious times. Deerfield Beach (FL): Health Communications, Inc; 2004.

[11] Griffith JL, Griffith ME. Encountering the sacred in psychotherapy: how to talk with people about their spiritual lives. New York: Guilford; 2002.

[12] Abernethy AD, Lancia JJ. Religion and the psychotherapeutic relationship: transference and counter transferential dimensions. J Psychother Pract Res 1998;7:281–9.

[13] Psychopathology Committee of the Group for the Advancement of Psychiatry. Reexamination of therapist self-disclosure. Psychiatr Serv 2001;52(11):1489–93.

[14] Peteet J. Therapeutic implications of worldview. In: Josephson A, Peteet J, editors. Handbook of spirituality and worldview in clinical practice. Washington, DC: American Psychiatric Publishing, Inc; 2004. p. 47–59.

[15] Post SP, Puchalski CM, Larson DB. Physicians and patient spirituality: professional boundaries, competency, and ethics. Ann Intern Med 2000;132(7):578–83.

[16] American Psychiatric Association, Committee on Religion and Psychiatry. Guidelines regarding possible conflict between psychiatrists' religious commitments and psychiatric practice. Am J Psychiatry 1990;147(4):542.

[17] Sexson S. Religious and spiritual assessment of the child and adolescent. Child Adolesc Psychiatr Clin N Am 2004;13:35–47.

[18] Koenig HG, Pritchett J. Religion and psychotherapy. In: Koenig HG, editor. Handbook of religion and mental health. San Diego (CA): Academic Press; 1988. p. 323–36.

[19] Sheehan W, Kroll J. Psychiatric patients' belief in general health factors and sin as causes of illness. Am J Psychiatry 1990;147:112–3.

[20] Peteet J. Doing the right thing: an approach to moral issues in mental health treatment. Washington, DC: American Psychiatric Publishing, Inc; 2004.

[21] Kendler KS, Gardner CO, Prescott CA. Religion, psychopathology, and substance abuse: a multimeasure, genetic-epidemiologic study. Am J Psychiatry 1997;154:322–9.

[22] Weaver AJ, Samford JA, Morgan V, et al. Research on religious variables in five major adolescent research journals: 1992 to 1996. J Nerv Ment Dis 2000;188:36–44.

[23] Hallfors D, Waller M, Bauer D, et al. Which comes first in adolescence—sex and drugs or depression? Am J Prev Med 2005;29:163–70.

[24] Studer M, Thornton A. Adolescent religiosity and contraceptive usage. J Marriage Fam 1987;49:117–28.

[25] Dell ML. Religious professionals and institutions: untapped resources for clinical care. Child Adolesc Psychiatr Clin N Am 2004;13:85–110.

[26] Allport GW, Ross JM. Personal religious orientation and prejudice. J Pers Soc Psychol 1967;5:432–43.

[27] Richards PS, Bergin AE. Handbook of psychotherapy and religious diversity. Washington, DC: American Psychological Association; 2000.

[28] Rizzuto AM. The birth of the living god. A psychoanalytic inquiry. Chicago: University of Chicago Press; 1979.

[29] Freud S. Future of an illusion (1927). In: Strachey J, editor, The standard edition of the complete psychological works of Sigmund Freud, Vol. 20. London: Hogarth Press; 1962. p. 5–56.

[30] Kleinman A. Rethinking psychiatry: from cultural category to personal experience. New York: Free Press; 1988. p. 86–7.

How to Pass the Psychiatry Oral Board Examination

Jack Krasuski, MD

The American Board of Psychiatry and Neurology (ABPN) Psychiatry Part II Examination (the "oral boards") is among the most challenging exams in all of medicine. The pass rate for the oral boards has hovered around 55% to 60% for years and remains lower than in other medical specialties [1,2]. Indeed, the oral boards have become an all-too-painful "rite of passage" for young psychiatrists.

Residency programs have designed innovative mock examinations to help candidates feel more comfortable and to be better prepared. If you have an interest in designing such a program, details are available [3]. The recent change in exam format, which I'll be discussing in this article, may raise the pass rate. Nevertheless, make no mistake, this exam remains difficult and requires extensive preparation to pass.

I was asked to write this article by the editor of this issue of the *Psychiatric Clinics of North America* because I have spent much of my professional career trying to help psychiatrists pass these boards, and to do so with the least pain and most enjoyment possible–for the learning that can occur in the preparation process can be both valuable and enjoyable if the candidate has the appropriate attitude.

Let me elaborate on my last comment, that some may find puzzling. For most people the boards occur at a crucial and exciting time in their careers–the early postgraduate years–when we are establishing our practices, forging our identities, and working with substantially less supervision. It is a wonderful time to consolidate what we have learned during our residencies and to push ourselves to further improve our clinical skills so as to optimize our ability to help others. Moreover, "the move out of the nest" can be a bit harrowing, and with a sound, concerted effort at intensively securing our clinical acumen, we can emerge with a good deal more confidence, which helps us–not only to provide better care–but to make our jobs a good deal more fun. Confidence in our skills is an immense gift.

Consequently, I urge you to view your preparation for the boards, to be not only an important task for passing them, but as a uniquely rich chance to

E-mail address: jk@blueti.com

0193-953X/07/$ – see front matter
doi:10.1016/j.psc.2007.02.006

become a more skilled and mature clinician. It really is a great opportunity for advancement of clinical skill.

The source of the insights that follow is based on my experience of personally training over 400 psychiatry oral board candidates each year. Keep in mind, that all of the following suggestions are merely my own opinions and are not coming from the ABPN. In the interests of full disclosure, and to give some sense of my credibility to write an article that can help you to pass the boards, here are a few facts about my qualifications:

I derive income from preparing psychiatrists for the oral boards and other board exams. The large numbers of psychiatrists I train gives me a "down-in-the-trenches" understanding of the errors that candidates make and how to most quickly prepare for the boards [4].

I failed my oral boards twice before finally (hallelujah!) passing on my third attempt. I believe I richly deserved to fail my first two exams and concur with my examiners' decisions.

I have never worked for nor am I associated with the ABPN. I hope the reader will find my independent point of view refreshing.

My goal in this article is to write a no-nonsense, nitty gritty, primer on how to pass the oral boards. To do so, we will cover the following areas:

1. Description of the oral board format
2. Information on what knowledge-base areas are covered and how best to prepare yourself to have the knowledge base you will need
3. Tips for passing the 30-minute interview format
4. Tips for passing the 60-minute vignette format

In each of the sections I will also suggest books that may be of particular value (and explain why). I know you have little time to read, and I'd like to give you a heads-up on where that time may be best spent.

PART I. THE FORMAT OF THE ORAL BOARDS

The oral board exam consists of two examination sections: the patient interview examination and the vignette examination.

The patient interview lasts approximately 30 minutes and is immediately followed by a 30-minute session with examiners during which the candidate presents the entire case and responds to examiner questions.

The vignette exam, instituted in May 2006, lasts approximately 60 minutes and consists of four vignettes, three written and one video, each presented at a separate station. The candidate has each vignette read to him and observes the video and, in each case, responds to a series of questions based on the data presented in the written or video vignette.

An excellent book (which I feel certain is being updated to the new board format) in which you can gain a more realistic understanding and feeling for what the board experience is really like, was written by Morrison and Munoz [1] and carries the title, *Boarding Time: The Psychiatry Candidate's New Guide to the*

Part II of the ABPN Examination. The title almost makes it sound like fun, doesn't it? Concise and well-written, it is well worth your money and time. Pay particular attention to their descriptions of how to prepare for the experience both mentally and through practice.

PART II. THE NEEDED KNOWLEDGE BASE AND HOW TO GET IT

Put succinctly, deficits in the knowledge base include deficits both in the *Diagnostic and Statistical Manual,* fourth edition TR (*DSM-IV-TR*) diagnostic criteria and in the treatment and management of patients. In this section we will look at tips in the following three areas: (1) *DSM-IV-TR* diagnostic criteria, (2) psychotherapeutic knowledge, and (3) core treatment planning knowledge.

How to Master the DSM-IV-TR Diagnostic Criteria

With the new vignette format, candidates are exposed to four vignette cases, thus increasing the breadth of diagnostic knowledge that can be assessed. To be blunt, candidates need to review diagnostic criteria more thoroughly.

Since attempting to read through and memorize the *DSM-IV-TR* can be boring, and thus difficult to attend to, I provide this recommendation: when studying the *DSM-IV-TR*, the candidate should translate each criterion into question form, as if querying a patient for the presence of that symptom. This increases the degree of mental processing required during the study period and thus increases attentiveness to the task. The candidate also gains practice in generating queries from diagnostic criteria.

With Which Psychotherapies Should Candidates Be Familiar?

Candidates, at a minimum, should be able to articulate the basics of the following forms of psychotherapies:

Psychodynamic therapy
Cognitive behavioral therapy (CBT) including techniques such as cognitive restructuring and exposure-response prevention
Dialectical behavioral therapy (DBT)
Supportive therapy
Psychosocial rehabilitation programs
Chemical dependence rehabilitation (eg, motivation enhancement therapy, relapse prevention therapy)

In the above list, I wish to highlight chemical dependence rehabilitation (addiction treatment) because that is the area of greatest weakness for the largest number of candidates. In particular, candidates should know that 12-Step Programs are adequate interventions only for some patients but not for most and are NOT the same treatment intervention as a rehabilitation program, which incorporates a case manager and cognitive behaviorally–based interventions.

With regard to preparatory reading, you might enjoy a quick perusal of my monograph, "Lightning Review of the Psychotherapies" [5].

Knowledge About Treatment Interventions: What to Know and What Not to Know

It goes without saying that you must be well-grounded in key biologic therapies—especially psychopharmacology—as well as core psychosocial interventions. The logical question arises, "How much do I need to know?"

Once again, I recommend viewing your educational review for the boards as an opportunity for optimizing your clinical knowledge so that you can provide even better care for your patients in the years to come. Accomplish this task and you will have prepared well for the boards. From an operational level one can view the task as follows: the psychiatrist must be able to convey sufficient information to the patient about each and every intervention prescribed by the psyhiatrist so that the patient is in a position to give valid informed consent.

The psychiatrist must know the indications and benefits of the intervention, the potential adverse effects of the intervention, the alternate treatments available, and the risks and benefits of the alternative interventions. In addition, a competent psychiatrist should know enough about the practicalities and underlying concepts of the treatment to be able to sensitively explain the treatment to the patient and the patient's family. The psychiatrist also should know enough to respond to the common questions that patients and families may have about that form of treatment.

I will use electroconvulsive therapy (ECT) as an example, since most psychiatrists do not administer this form of treatment, yet must competently include it in their armamentarium. So, how much does a psychiatrist need to know to prescribe ECT and to obtain informed consent from a patient? This is my view:

> The psychiatrist need NOT know the dose of methylhexitol or whichever other induction agent is given the patient,or perhaps even that methylhexitol is an induction agent.
> The psychiatrist need NOT know the exact voltage/current settings of the ECT machine.
> The psychiatrist need NOT be competent in personally administering ECT.

The psychiatrist does need to know this:

> The indications for ECT, including, for instance, that it may be particularly apt as a treatment for pregnant women with severe mania.
> The adverse effects of ECT, including that there is 1 in 10,000 to 1 in 50,000 risk of death with each treatment.
> The conceptual basis of ECT's efficacy (eg, being able to explain to the patient that the electrical current induces a short seizure in the brain lasting less than a minute, and that it is the seizure that, for unclear reasons, has mood-stabilizing effects).

The outline of the procedure (eg, that patients are "asleep" under general anesthesia and that they receive a "muscle relaxant" so that they do not sustain injury during the seizure; that they must take nothing by mouth from midnight and must have someone drive them home following the procedure, if it is done as an outpatient procedure).

With regard to knowledge-based preparation, if you want to read just one book, I really like Nathan Strahl's *Clinical Study Guide for the Oral Boards in Psychiatry*, second edition [6]. It is concise and well written, and it represents a great "one-stop-shop" for getting the core knowledge base you need to pass the boards. Another nice book, if you want just a little more beef is *Tasman's Pocket Companion to Accompany Psychiatry* [7]. It is an easy-to-read, condensed version of his major textbook on psychiatry, and it almost as if it were written to prepare one for the boards, with concise sections on *DSM-IV* diagnostic criteria, descriptive psychopathology, psychotherapies, psychopharmacology, and other treatments.

PART III. TIPS ON PASSING THE PATIENT INTERVIEW EXAMINATION

In many respects the patient interview is the most daunting and intimidating part of the examination for examinees. It does not necessarily have to be so, although don't get me wrong, it is filled with pressures (I failed twice, so I know of what I speak). With time, and in helping so many people to pass the boards, I have come to realize how much successful completion depends on attitude. In this regard, fear is clearly not the desired attitude. Choking is not limited to sporting events.

In the second edition of his book, *Psychiatric Interviewing, the Art of Understanding*, Shea [8] provides a useful appendix dedicated to tips on passing the oral boards. His sage advice can help the examinee avoid unnecessary anxiety:

"One of the biggest hurdles I find, with clinicians having problems with the Boards, arises from an unnecessarily intense fear of the Boards themselves, often generated by a false belief. This anxiety-provoking belief sounds one way or another something like the following statement, ''The Boards are extremely difficult and artificial. They don't look like any type of clinical interview that I do.''

"Don't say this to yourself, because it is very anxiety producing and suggests that the examinee is being tested on a technique that is unfamiliar. This concept is indeed a frightening thought. Avoid it—it is very counterproductive."

"But there is a more important reason to avoid this belief, other than that it is counterproductive. It is patently false. You have successfully performed a similar 30-minute interview many times in your training, under extremely difficult circumstances, and you have done it well. You have performed this type of interview when you have been ''beat tired,'' harried, and under incredible time pressures. You have done this style of interview successfully many times, when an error does not result in someone failing a test but can result in someone losing his or her life. You have successfully and gracefully done this interview many times, because you have done a very similar interview every single time that you have been "on call." You see, in many respects the "Board Interview" is an emergency room interview with a few extras."

"When you enter the interview room, don't focus on passing a test. Focus on doing a good clinical interview, much like you have done scores of times in the emergency room. Tell yourself, "I've done this before and I know how to do it." Do a good clinical interview, and you will have done a good "Board Interview."

"The APBN is trying to ensure that practicing psychiatrists are safe and can soundly perform key clinical skills such as interviewing, case formulation, and treatment planning. They are not trying to see if you can do a comprehensive 60-minute intake in 30 minutes. The Board is attempting to determine whether the interviewer can gather a reasonable database in a 30-minute time period that results in a sound formulation and disposition. They do not expect you to do the impossible, but they do expect you to appropriately structure the patient toward giving pertinent information. In a nutshell they want to see if examinees are facile at engagement, practical in choosing areas to explore, and safe in judgement. These skills are exactly the ones that you have used numerous times in the emergency room."

Savor these words by Shea. Read these paragraphs over and over, until the wisdom sinks into your bones. It really is true that, except for a few small modifications, you already have done this type of interview and done it well. Relax.

Moreover, I think I have a variety of tips and strategies that can help you navigate this interview segment of the oral boards successfully. The tips can be arranged in the following categories, each of which we will take a look at:

Types of patient you are likely to encounter
Logistics of the format
Importance of exam prep
How to practice the interview
How to practice presenting the history and treatment formulation
The style of the interview as in the "good enough" interview
How to avoid big mistake #1–the sketchy interview
How to avoid big mistake #2–ignoring psychologic factors and the psychodynamics of the interview itself

What Types of Patients Can You Expect to Interview?

The sites at which the actual exams occur invariably include a university hospital and clinic and a Veterans Administration medical center. The sites also frequently include a state psychiatric hospital and at least one community hospital and clinic. The interviewee-patient may be receiving treatment in either an inpatient or outpatient setting.

Often patients from specialty clinics are recruited as interviewees. Therefore it is possible that a candidate will interview a patient from, for instance, an eating disorders clinic, a women's clinic, or a dialectical behavioral therapy program.

Patients may be high-functioning individuals, such as attorneys, college professors, and mental health workers, or conversely, lower-functioning individuals with severe major mental illness as well as homeless individuals residing in area shelters. Hospital units from which patients are drawn include forensic units and other long-term units in which patients remain hospitalized for years or even decades.

The Logistics of the Live Patient Interview Examination

On arriving at the examination site, the candidate is ushered to a waiting room where he or she waits with the other candidates. At the appointed time the candidates' names are called sequentially. The called candidate steps out of the waiting room and meets his two examiners. The examiners then walk with the candidate to the assigned room where the patient is waiting.

Once in the room, the candidate's goal is to seat himself or herself across from the patient and wait as the examiners seat themselves. If the chair is not positioned conveniently, the candidate can reposition it. It is unnecessary, however, to start rearranging the furniture for the sake of taking control or for the sake of having something to do. The candidate's behavior should be that of a clinical psychiatrist conducting a diagnostic interview with a new patient.

The Importance of Adequate Examination Preparation

Failing performances on the oral boards may be related either to deficits in the candidate's knowledge base or to deficits in observable skills such as interviewing, presenting, and thinking on one's feet. Of the two deficits, I believe that candidates fail more frequently because of deficits in observable skills as opposed to a lack of knowledge.

You must be absolutely clear that the oral board exam is a performance. As performers, candidates are in the same category as dancers, musicians, athletes, and soldiers. Given this fact, it is critical that candidates should prepare for the oral boards not only by brushing up on the clinically relevant knowledge base, but also by practicing board-style interviews, case presentations, and question-and-answer sessions. There are three keys to passing the interview section of the boards: (1) Practice, (2) Practice, and (3) Practice. Moreover, the more realistic the practice sessions are, the more learning and desensitization are achieved [3,9].

How to Practice the Interview

To do well, candidates are advised to practice board-style interviews and case presentations. Many candidates consistently undermine the power of their practice interviews by taking effectiveness-sapping shortcuts. Here are tips on doing it right [10].

1. Practice 30-minute diagnostic interviews and do not take a moment longer. I've done hundreds of practice board-style interviews over the years to keep my skills sharp. This is what I've learned—doing an interview that is 32 or 33 minutes long is very different from doing one that is the required 30 minutes. (In the examination, however, the 30-minute time is approximate. Oral

board examiners may end the interview slightly earlier or, rarely, permit the candidate to continue for somewhat longer. These small deviations from the norm should not be taken as a reason not to prepare for the normal allotted time.) By doing the interview right, the candidate develops procedural or "body" memory for doing it just that way. On a personal note, for me, the challenge in conducting competent board-style interviews is fitting all the interview regions into the allotted time. I chronically run overtime and I need to practice repeatedly in order to adjust my pace to the 30-minute interview.

2. Do NOT use your own patients in practice interviews. The dynamic between a physician and patient in the process of establishing an ongoing therapeutic relationship differs from the dynamic between a physician whose interaction with the patient is limited to a single diagnostic interview and differs even more when the single interview, as on the board exam does not involve a formal clinical provider-patient relationship.

3. Call a colleague to get permission to interview his or her patients with whom you do not have a physician-patient relationship. Explain the purpose of the interview to the prospective interviewees and obtain their oral agreement. (Some clinics have policies that obligate you to obtain written consent when interviewing patients from their clinics for training purposes.) Depending on the policies and/or expectations, offer to pay the interviewee $10 to $20 for each interview. Since you're there at the clinic, conduct two or three successive interviews to speed the establishment of your "body memory" for conducting board-style interviews.

4. It is preferable to have a colleague mock examine you. If you can not get this in place, do NOT let it stop you from doing the practice board-style interviews. I cannot stress enough how important practice interviews are, even without an observer/examiner.

5. If you DO have a colleague who will mock exam you, you will benefit because it adds another layer of realism to your practice session. Even if your colleague has not taken the oral boards or has taken them but is not a good assessor of your performance, just having someone observing your performance is effective in helping you desensitize to being observed and judged. (By the way, most colleagues will tell you that you "did fine." Do not necessarily take their word on it. Most people do not know what to look for. Nevertheless, the benefit lies in helping you desensitize to being observed and judged.)

6. Do NOT be shy asking for help. If colleagues are not readily available in your home town, strongly consider contacting your former residency director. Most residency directors are willing and even eager to help recent graduates. Your success reflects on them and their program. Again, there is no shame in asking for help. You are not an expert in the oral boards and your ignorance of the process or of the expectations for your performance does not reflect negatively on you.

How to Practice Presenting the History, Case Formulation, and Treatment Plan

Shea [8] makes the pithy point that, unlike the 30-minute board-style interview, which is similar to the 30-minute interview that you have done many times before in an emergency room, case presentation may very well be something that you have seldom done. Equally importantly, you may have received previous little training in how to do it well. In short, this is one part of the oral exam that most of us do not do routinely in our daily practices. Consequently, it is imperative that you practice presenting. There is a definite art to doing it effectively. It really is a performance skill. Rightly or wrongly, examiners may make a quick decision on your skill level based on how fluid and organized your presentation is. As in social situations, first impressions count.

My advice is simple: practice doing your interview and then immediately allow yourself only a minute to prepare your presentation and proceed to provide a succinct presentation to a colleague, or, if no one is available, in front of a mirror. If you make a mistake, do NOT stop. Practice covering your mistake gracefully, exactly as you would in the examination room. Also be aware that during your presentation, some examiners may stop you to ask a question. Never look flustered or irritated at the interruption. Simply field the question gracefully and then proceed with your presentation. Shea [8] describes a number of other tips for quickly organizing the presentation and for giving it fluidly. Space limitations prevent a discussion of those tips here, but I urge you to take a look at them.

The "Good Enough" Interview

What type of interview should I do? The answer is a "good enough" interview that would allow you to make a safe disposition and treatment plan if you only had 30 minutes with a patient, much as you would do in an emergency room. If you do so, then you will have done a "good enough" interview to pass the boards as well. Candidates get into trouble when they try to do a perfect 60-minute interview in 30 minutes. It can't be done.

The interview is only 30 minutes long. To be blunt, something has to give. In 30 minutes even an excellent interviewer cannot obtain full detail in every area of psychopathology. A 30-minute initial psychiatric diagnostic interview allows only 15 to 17 minutes for straight diagnostic interviewing. The rest of the time should be devoted to obtaining other pertinent psychiatric information such as social history, family history, lethality assessment, conducting a screening cognitive assessment, and responding to the patient's questions or concerns as they arise. In a good board-style interview, you will even, at times, take a minute or two to pursue a more psychodynamically-informed line of questioning as deemed relevant.

From watching literally hundreds of interviews, I have found that a common error candidates make is to devote too MUCH time to one particular area of psychopathology or diagnosis. A common candidate profile is the "diagnostic perfectionist." This type of candidate asks every last symptom criterion on every single syndrome that is present (or could be present) and follows this by evaluating the temporal relationships among all the symptoms. Such a perfectionistic–dare I say obsessive-compulsive–candidate usually is usually positively stunned when time is up, only then realizing that he or she has obtained little or no medical, social, and family history nor have they conducted even a cursory screening cognitive exam.

The difficulty some perfectionistic candidates encounter is that it is emotionally difficult to "let go and move on" before a complete diagnostic picture is established. Even though perfectionistic candidates may have an intellectual understanding of the need to pace themselves and even have a watch on the clipboard to guide their use of time, they are unable emotionally to tolerate the sense of a lack of completion. That lack of completion, however, is the feeling perfectionistic candidates must learn to tolerate to give themselves adequate time to pursue other areas of crucial interest. Note that it is also the skill that a talented emergency room psychiatrist must have in order to function effectively in a hectic emergency department. I have described other problematic "styles" of interviewing, akin to the "diagnostic perfectionist" in my free e-book, *12 Mistakes That Will Sink Your Oral Boards and How to Avoid Them* [11].

A note of warning to candidates who believe that the social history is optional and of second-level interest. I emphatically say, "Not true!" Exactly as in the real world of a clinic or emergency room, if an examinee only understands a patient's psychopathology, without understanding the patient's station in life, stresses, and underlying concerns, then the interviewer understands little about the most important thing—the person beneath the diagnostic label. Consequently, the interviewer will not be in a position to present an individualized and nuanced treatment plan relevant to the unique human being whom he or she just interviewed. Trust me on this one, examiners do not like this trait in a candidate—big time.

So what approach should a candidate take to avoid the curse of perfectionism?

Three levels of detail
Because the oral board interview is brief, not all areas of psychopathology can be assessed thoroughly. The candidate, however, is expected to delve deeply enough into the patient's psychopathology to establish a working diagnosis. One approach to resolving this dilemma is to assess different areas of psychopathology to various degrees of precision.

Highest level of detail
Assess the chief complaint/working diagnosis with the highest level of detail. For instance, if the patient gives as a chief complaint, "I'm in treatment for schizophrenia," the candidate should plan on conducting a highly detailed assessment of psychotic symptoms. This means querying Schneidarian first-rank types of delusions and hallucinations. If the patient does not endorse "hearing voices when no one is around," the candidate should notice the discrepancy between the patient's self-reported diagnosis and the denial of auditory hallucinations.

This discrepancy may mean that the patient truly never experienced auditory hallucinations, that the patient is lying (perhaps in response to command hallucinations telling the patient to deny the presence of voices), or that the patient has a different understanding of the hallucinatory experience than the question suggests (there is a miscommunication between interviewer and patient).

For instance, the patient may believe he or she hears voices only when people ARE around. The voices may be experienced as coming from the air ducts connecting the apartment next door or from neighbors whispering about the patient from their gangways as the patient walks down the street to return home. In both cases the patient may truthfully deny "hearing voices when no one is around," because the phrasing of the question did not reflect accurately his or her experience of the phenomenon.

In such a case, I recommend following up with questions such as, "Do you ever find that people are whispering about you?" and, "Do you ever receive telepathic messages or intercept radio waves?" and, "Do spirits or other beings ever speak to you?" Only after such a more detailed query can a candidate validly report to the examiners that the patient denied presence of auditory hallucinations.

Always keep in mind that a personality disorder, such as borderline personality, may be the major problem and focus of care, in which case a thorough exploration is required.

Moderate level of detail
Assess the syndromes highly comorbid with the chief complaint/working diagnosis with a moderate level of detail. Continuing the above example, if a candidate believes that the patient's working diagnosis will turn out to be a form of schizophrenia, he or she should assess other possible disorders in the differential diagnosis that also could cause psychotic symptoms with some care, such as mood disorders, substance abuse disorders, delusional disorders, and organic causes of psychosis.

Lowest level of detail
You should plan on conducting a review of psychiatric symptoms that briefly covers the areas of psychopathology that either have not been raised spontaneously by the patient nor yet assessed by the candidate because they did not appear to be related to the chief complaint or to be highly comorbid with it. Don't forget that Axis II process may need to be tapped lightly.

With regard to strategically fitting in all the other pertinent topics for a board exam interview—a very brief cognitive examination, social history, family history, past psychiatric history, medical history, and suicide assessment—there are different strategies you can take, and I suggest you familiarize yourself with them so that you can flexibly adapt as the interview proceeds [1,8].

Avoiding Big Mistake #1—the "Sketchy Interview"
Earlier we reviewed the "perfectionistic interviewer" and I suggested how to avoid that problem. In addition, the opposite approach also may be lethal,

that is, an interview that is far too incomplete in diagnostic information. These are some of the ways the "sketch-artist" approach can occur:

The candidate who has a mistaken notion of the level of detail the examiners expect: The majority of examiners expect that the most likely diagnoses, and especially the working diagnosis, will be supported by an assessment of specific diagnostic criteria. Our "three levels of detail" from above apply. For instance, when a patient reports, "I've been depressed for 3 months. My mood is low, and I haven't been able to work," the candidate should follow up with, "What other symptoms of depression did you notice?" and then, if a major depressive episode has not yet been established, to follow that with assessment of other symptom criteria.

The candidate who is lulled into complacency by a talkative, easygoing patient: Some patients are overinclusive on details that do not advance the clinician's diagnostic understanding. Some candidates accept the patient's "chattiness" and only during the case presentation realize their dearth of specific diagnostic detail.

The candidate who finds it difficult to interrupt and redirect the patient when needed: Other candidates, especially those who were raised in more traditional cultures than the prevailing, more casual one in the United States, often find it difficult to interrupt patients because interruptions are considered rude and offensive. Although all candidates should minimize interrupting patients and avoid speaking over patients, some interruptions are necessary. The perspective to take is that the candidate is a professional who needs to obtain enough information to form a sensible professional judgment.

The candidate who stops the interview early with the mistaken notion that he or she has obtained all the information needed. For any candidate who, during the board exam is tempted to stop the interview before being told to do so by the examiners, I have one comment, "Plan on coming back. You WILL fail!" During our board review courses, never once have I witnessed a passing interview conducted by a participant who ended early. There simply are too many facts that can and should be obtained from even the most seemingly straightforward case to permit completion of a diagnostic interview in less than 30 minutes.

Avoiding Big Mistake #2—Ignoring Psychological Factors and the Psychodynamics of the Interview Itself

My "Beat The Boards!" Course participants often convey a sense of frustration at my strong focus on psychological issues, particularly what the significance is of specific patient behaviors or statements made to the interviewer during the interview itself. Such interpersonal dynamics are great grist for the mill to board examiners. They love to ask about such stuff. Let me share an example:

Dr. Bhatti (not his real name) interviews Ms. Begamy (not her real name). Dr. Bhatti is a rather heavy-set man who is quite anxious and is sweating profusely as he enters the examination room on a warm September day in Indianapolis. During the introduction phase, Ms. Begamy hands Dr. Bhatti a tissue to wipe his brow. He thanks her and continues orienting her to the interview process.

Ms. Begamy interrupts him in midsentence and asks if he is board certified. He says no and continues his incessant stream of questions. She interrupts again and, pointing in the direction of the two seated examiners, asks Dr. Bhatti if they are board certified. Flustered, Dr. Bhatti says he thinks so and then corrects himself, saying that of course they must be because they are examiners. That is the end of this exchange, and Dr. Bhatti conducts the rest of his interview without further occurrence.

When Dr. Bhatti begins to present the case, he reported to me that one of his examiners interrupted him almost immediately and asked what Dr. Bhatti made of the fact that Ms. Begamy handed him a tissue to wipe his brow. Dr. Bhatti became flustered and was unprepared to respond to such a question. He told me that he thought, "Can you just leave me alone and let me present the case!"

The answer is, "No." The examiners, wisely and expectedly, were highly interested in this exchange, wondering what the possible meanings and implications of the "here and now" interaction between the physician and the patient could mean. Indeed, in actual clinical practice, such an awareness and the subsequent corrective attention to the patient's concerns and anxieties might be critical for fostering a more effective engagement, gathering a more valid database, enhancing the patient's "buy-in" to medication recommendations, and even securing that a second appointment occurs.

The problems that candidates encounter when faced with psychologically meaningful patient behaviors during the interview (and with psychologically focused examiner questions after the interview) are several. First, many candidates do not understand their importance and thus do not attend to them. Second, even when candidates realize the need to attend to such communications, their performance anxiety interferes with their ability to maintain a broad awareness of these communications as they occur in real time during the interview. Third, even if candidates realize the need to attend to such psychologically meaningful behaviors and do so, they do not have the ability to articulate their observations and thus, often keep silent from fear of saying something that will "get me into trouble." Fourth, and this is for many psychiatrists, the foundational problem, is that so MANY psychiatrists have little to no training in developing a psychodynamic or, more broadly, a psychological understanding of their patients and the need for flexible approaches to their care dependent on their psychological quirks and proclivities.

Fortunately, several books can really help you to tackle these problems and prepare effectively for the interview section of the boards. Right off the bat, if you only have time to read one book on interviewing, I would begin with Shawn Shea's *Psychiatric Interviewing: the Art of Understanding*, second edition [8]. It covers all the bases mentioned previously, from *DSM-IV-TR* diagnosis to effective structuring and time-management, and is fun to read.

In addition, as I had stated earlier, preparing for the boards is a good way to prepare oneself to be a better clinician in ensuing years. Shea's book is a perfect example of this principle, for it is not just an interviewing primer, it is also a sophisticated exploration of advanced interviewing tips illustrated with vivid depictions of patients from actual clinical practice. With regard to avoiding Big Mistake #2, Shea provides a wealth of information concerning the psychological and psychodynamic aspects of the interview, including methods for "opening-up" reticent patients, "roping-in" wandering patients, handling awkward patient questions such as Dr. Bhatti encountered, and understanding and using nonverbal communication.

Another gem of a book, useful both for board preparation and growth as a clinician, is Carlat's *The Psychiatric Interview: a Practical Guide*, second edition [12]. Carlat, a noted expert on psychopharmacology, is also a gifted interviewer and writer. His book is filled with an array of great interviewing questions for uncovering *DSM-IV-TR* diagnoses and is written with a real sense of practicality. Finally, if you want a particularly sophisticated exploration of the psychodynamic aspects of the interview (yet another great bridge into advanced practice), you can't go wrong with the second edition of MacKinnon and colleagues' [13] classic text, *The Psychiatric Interview in Clinical Practice*.

PART IV: TIPS ON PASSING THE 60-MINUTE VIGNETTE EXAMINATION

In this section, we will cover the following key areas:

The logistics of the vignette examination
A comparison of the new vignette format with the old format
What type of questions that might be asked
Some special areas of knowledge base often focused upon in the vignette section (including consult-liaison issues, forensic concerns, information gleaned from the mental status, and interpersonal dynamics between the patient and the observed interviewer such as transference/countertransference issues)

The Logistics of the Vignette Exam

The new vignette examination replaced the 30-minute videotaped interview exam section beginning in May of 2006. The new vignette examination consists of four vignettes presented in a period of 60 minutes. Each vignette is presented by one examiner at a separate station. The candidate is given approximately 3 minutes to transfer between stations, which are located in separate rooms. That leaves the candidate approximately 12 minutes to review the vignette and respond to the examiner's queries.

Three vignettes are written and one is a video clip. The written vignettes are between 300 and 500 words in length and take about 3 minutes to read. The video clip is approximately 4 to 5 minutes in length.

Each written vignette has a primary area of focus, either diagnostic or treatment related. The video vignette presents a patient with either predominantly Axis I or Axis II psychopathology.

The New Vignette Format Compared with the 30-Minute Videotaped Format

The consensus among psychiatrists that I have spoken with, who have been examined using both the old-style 30-minute videotaped interview format and the new vignette format, seems to be a preference for the new format. The two most common positive comments I hear are (1) the new exam format no longer requires the candidate to generate an entire case presentation based on an interview the candidate did not conduct. Rather, the candidate now simply responds to one question at a time. (2) The exam is more guided and thus decreases uncertainty and anxiety among most candidates. Also, the new format places a greater emphasis on one's knowledge base as compared to one's ability to perform. This may particularly benefit international medical graduates, who often have a strong knowledge base.

On the negative side, some candidates report that the new format felt fast-paced and mentally draining. Also, with four separate cases replacing a single long case, the ability of the ABPN to test multiple areas of knowledge is greatly increased. Candidates feel like there is "no place to hide." By the way, this probably means it is a more valid test of clinical skills. Now more than ever, a candidate must be prepared in every aspect of psychiatric diagnosis and care.

Questions You Might Encounter in the Vignette and Video-clip Exam

To provide you with a sampling of the type of questions you might encounter in this segment of the boards, let me take a typical 300- to 500-word vignette and radically shorten it to three sentences, just to give us a basis for seeing where the questions might come from. Imagine the following synopsis is about 400 words longer and that you have just had it read to you:

> A 50-year-old woman, bedridden, living with her daughter, believes her food and tapwater are being poisoned. She is distrustful of men. She has a history of multiple neuroleptic use for short periods of time and is now referred to you by her internist.

Here are questions that examiners might come up with from such a case history:

1. Doctor, how would you address the patient's noncompliance?
2. What is your medical treatment plan? What meds will you start her on?
3. What psychotherapy would you recommend for her?
4. If the patient were diagnosed with breast cancer, what would you recommend to the surgeons?
5. What type of social treatment will you consider?
6. If the patient's daughter moved to another state, how would you alter your treatment plan for the patient?

Knowledge Base Areas That May Be of Particular Focus in the Vignette Exam

The new exam format permits a broad assessment of psychiatrists' competencies. Below are the areas that are currently receiving much greater emphasis. I describe each and give recommendations. By the way, these areas can also can come up in the questioning following your 30-minute patient interview, indeed, mental status questions almost always do. The areas of increased emphasis are:

Consult-liaison issues
Forensic issues
Mental status exam items
Interpersonal functioning, including transference-countertransference issues

Consult-liaison issues

As exemplified by our vignette synopsis from above, vignettes of patients with medical comorbidities such as cancer, renal failure, and hepatic insufficiency are common. This focus requires that candidates become more familiar with the effects of medical illnesses and medical treatments, including medications, on psychiatric conditions.

For instance, the vignette example is of a patient who has a psychotic disorder and who, the candidate is later told, has been diagnosed with breast cancer and is now awaiting surgery. The question, "What would you tell the surgeons?" is phrased broadly, purposely not suggesting a particular focus or boundaries of the response. In this case, the response would likely include a consideration of:

Whether the patient's antipsychotic medication(s) should be discontinued during the time of surgery
What alternative or additional medications or treatments should be considered
What behavioral problems can be anticipated, given the patient's psychiatric diagnosis
What specific issues the surgeons should be educated about

Forensic issues

Another area of increased focus is on forensic issues. All of the following can be considered fair game for examiner questions:

Treatment contracts
Informed consent and its exceptions
Confidentiality and its limits
Mandated reporting of child abuse and elder neglect
HIV disclosure guidelines
Duty to warn and duty to protect
Patient termination and patient abandonment

For instance, a vignette may present a young mother with acute decompensation who is the primary provider for her infant daughter. One of the concerns the candidate needs to recognize, and for which interventions must be recommended, regards the risk at which the infant is placed due to her mother's decompensation.

The candidate should recognize that he or she is a mandated reporter and would need to notify child protective services. Further, the candidate should recognize that removing the child from the mother's care, even temporarily, can be traumatic for the mother and that education and support may be indicated. The patient's rapport with and trust of the clinician also may be placed in jeopardy. Recognition of this may lead the candidate to address this issue directly with the patient whom he is about to report.

Mental status exam

There are only two forms of data that a candidate can obtain from the video clip and that is what he or she heard and observed. From my experience training candidates in responding to the video format, the candidates' observations are often inadequate. In fact, the shortcomings in the visual observation of videotaped patients are so frequent and so severe that I regard them as an example of an inherent limitation in our brain's ability to simultaneously process auditory and visual information that is accentuated under conditions of stress. Bottom line, you need to practice watching short videotaped interview segments and also practice how to describe the patient's mental status as seen on the video excerpt.

My recommendation is that on the video clip, candidates write as few notes as possible while, with conscious intent, keep scanning every aspect of the patient as seen on the screen. In addition, when preparing for the exam, candidates should carefully review the key concepts behind the mental status and the correct clinical descriptors that should be used in writing or describing a mental status. Also review what types of physical and psychiatric pathology might be suggested by specific mental status abnormalities.

As one common example of inadequate preparation on the mental status exam whenever a patient displays abnormalities in thought processes, the only descriptors I invariably hear from candidates are that the patient is "circumstantial" or "tangential," even when the patient is nothing of the sort, but, in fact is "overinclusive" or "perseverative" or shows signs of "poverty of thought content."

The way I characterize this problem is, "You don't see what you don't know" by which I convey that a phenomenon for which one does not have a specific term in mind is either not perceived, misperceived, or mischaracterized. My simple advice is that every oral board candidate carefully review the items and terms used when conducting a mental status exam. The chapter in Shea's book [8] on the mental status–its terms and implications–is excellent and all the review you will need.

Here are just a few more of the common items frequently missed that candidates should be closely looking for:

> Scanning the face for dysmorphisms and other anatomic or neurological abnormalities: if for example, the patient had the stigmata of fetal alcohol syndrome, would the candidate be able to detect it?

Observing the face, trunk, and limbs for disturbances in movement: Is range of motion full and movement fluid, or are there signs of rigidity? Are there any dyskinesias, and if so, what kind? Are there any tics, stereotypies, or mannerisms? (Of course, the candidate should at this point have reviewed, understood, and recognized the phenomena of tics, stereotypies, and mannerisms.)

Observing the patient's appearance: What is the body habitus? Is the patient obese or cachectic? Is grooming adequate, or is the patient disheveled or wearing odd clothes or makeup?

Listening to the patient's voice: Is the voice husky or raspy, or is a cough present? These are signs frequently present in smokers and could indicate various medical ailments.

Interpersonal dynamics occurring between the interviewer and the patient on the video excerpt

The video clips have as their focus either Axis I or Axis II psychopathology. Especially on the Axis II focused video clips, evidence of interpersonal functioning is stressed, including the transference and countertransference reactions between physician and patient.

Transference refers to the patient's emotional and behavioral reactions toward the interviewer. Countertransference refers to the clinician's emotional and behavioral reactions to the patient.

Here is what the ABPN tells us to attend to:

"Describe the patient's interaction with the interviewer and/or the pattern of relationships described in the video clip. Identify pertinent nonverbal communication and behavior demonstrated by the patient and the interviewer." (ABPN.com)

How do you approach transference and countertransference even if you don't feel comfortable in this area? Here is a simplified three-step approach to get you started:

Step 1: "Describe the behavior": Focus on the patient's behaviors toward the interviewer, without attempting to infer their meaning.

Step 2: "The transference step": Discuss how the patient's observed interpersonal behaviors are (1) likely to generalize to the patient's interactions with his or her entire treatment team and to important others in the patient's life and (2) what the implications this could have for the patient's treatment.

Step 3: "The countertransference step": Describe your reactions to the patient and how these reactions could affect your approach to the patient if you were the treating clinician. Remember that your reactions are likely to be the type of reactions that many other clinicians also would have. You are the stand-in for every other psychiatrist, mental health clinician, and even adult authority figure. Focus especially on how your possible emotional and behavioral reactions could derail or undermine the patient's treatment and how you would prevent this problem from happening.

How to Master Treatment Presentations and the Fielding of Questions Regarding Treatment

Serious knowledge deficits are often present in the area of treatment and management. Candidates should familiarize themselves with two categories of knowledge when it comes to treatment and management:

1. Information about each treatment intervention, whether the intervention is a medication (or other somatic treatment) or a form of psychotherapy (or other psychosocial intervention)
2. Treatment algorithms

The books I mentioned earlier on knowledge base should be adequate for your preparation here.

In the area of treatment, a common line of questioning by examiners might proceed as follows: You will be asked to present a biopsychosocial treatment plan. Whichever intervention you present first, you may be requested to describe it in a fair degree of detail. For instance, if the intervention is a medication such as divalproex sodium, you might be asked to discuss any work-up required prior to starting the medication, the starting dose, the target dose, potential adverse effects, possible drug-drug interactions, dose adjustments due to hepatic or renal insufficiency, and any follow-up assessments needed based on the patient's continued use of the medication.

A candidate who, for example, recommends prescribing divalproex sodium to a female patient of childbearing age who does not discuss the need for a pregnancy test and use of adequate birth control will probably be prompted to do so by the examiner (ie, given a chance to recognize the deficit in the recommended work-up). If the candidate does not pick up on this clue, that candidate may be failed for recommending a treatment without adequately assessing and protecting the patient.

After responding to the examiner's satisfaction regarding the initial treatment intervention, the next examiner statement is likely to be something like, "What if that medication, at that dose, didn't work. What would you do next?" The examiner is requesting that you proceed down a treatment algorithm, each time asking you, "If that intervention didn't work, what would you do next?" Thus, you should prepare by reviewing individual treatments and their treatment algorithms.

SUMMARY

I hope you enjoyed this article, and I also hope that it helps you to pass your oral boards. I firmly believe that having a sound outline and strategy, as presented in this article, can go a long way toward optimizing the power of your practice and readings as you prepare for this important rite of passage. Remember that everything you are studying can help you to provide better care. Keep in mind the ultimate mission—helping others—and the time spent in your board preparations can be surprisingly enjoyable, very rewarding, and much more likely to result in success. Good luck!

References

[1] Morrison J, Munoz RA. Boarding time: the psychiatry candidate's new guide to the part II of the ABPN examination. 3rd edition. Washington, DC: American Psychiatric Press Inc.; 2003.

[2] Moran M. New ABPN Executive Sees Big Changes for Board Exam. Psychiatric News 2006;41(10):10.

[3] Shea SC, Rancurello M. Faculty and resident response to an innovative mock board. Acad Psychiatry 1989;13:137–43.

[4] The Blue Tower Institute. Beat the Boards Course. Available at: www.beattheboards.com directed by Jack Krasuski, M.D., based in Lyons, Illinois.

[5] Krasuski J. Lightning review of the psychotherapies. Lyons (IL): Blue Tower Institute LLC; 2005–06.

[6] Strahl N. Clinical study guide for the oral boards in psychiatry. 2nd edition. Washington, DC: American Psychiatric Publishing, Inc.; 2005.

[7] Tasman A, Kay J, Lieberman J. Pocket companion to accompany psychiatry. Philadelphia: W.B. Saunders Company; 1998.

[8] Shea SC. Psychiatric interviewing the art of understanding. 2nd edition. Philadelphia: W.B. Saunders Company; 1998.

[9] Krasuski J. The ultimate step-by-step guide to the psychiatric oral board interview; 2004.

[10] Krasuski J. Special report: procrastinator proof oral board preparation. Lyons (IL): Blue Tower Institute LLC; 2005.

[11] Krasuski J. 12 mistakes that will sink your oral boards & how to avoid them. [e-book]. Lyons (IL): Blue Tower Institute LLC; 2002–05.

[12] Carlat DJ. The psychiatric interview: a practical guide. 2nd edition. New York: Lippincott Williams & Wilkins; 2004.

[13] MacKinnon RA, Michels RM, Buckley PJ. The psychiatric interview in clinical practice. 2nd edition. Washington, DC: American Psychiatric Publishing, Inc.; 2006.

Part II

Favorite Interviewing Tips from Those

Who "Wrote the Book"

My Favorite Tips from the "Clinical Interviewing Tip of the Month" Archive

Shawn Christopher Shea, MD[a,b,*]

[a]Training Institute for Suicide Assessment and Clinical Interviewing (TISA), 1502 Route 123 North, Stoddard, NH 03464, USA
[b]Dartmouth Medical School, Hanover, NH, USA

After launching the Website for the Training Institute for Suicide Assessment and Clinical Interviewing (TISA) in 1999, I have had the pleasure of editing a monthly feature of the TISA Website entitled the "Interviewing Tip of the Month" [1]. These interviewing gems are supplied by visitors to the Website or by participants in my workshops. Each month I choose a favorite tip for posting and then add the past month's tip to the "Tip Archive." (At last count there were more than 80 tips in the archive). On the Website I always provide a "TISA Description of the Problem" that frames the interviewing problem that the tip addresses and a "TISA Clinical Caveat" that further frames the use of the tip or adds another interviewing suggestion. These sections also are included below.

I have learned so much from the tips, which visitors to the Website shared, that it sparked the idea for this section of the *Psychiatric Clinics of North America*. I thought to myself, "What would happen if I asked the greatest interviewers of our time to provide two or three of their favorite interviewing tips?" That answer, as further articles show, is quite remarkable.

Before touching base with the masters, here are some of the outstanding clinical interviewing tips, provided by front-line clinicians from around the world, that started the phenomenon. Below are eight of my favorite tips from the "Interviewing Tip of the Month."

INTERVIEWING TIP #1: SENSITIVELY UNCOVERING THE CLIENT'S WORK HISTORY—PITFALLS AND SOLUTIONS
Description of the Problem
Many aspects of taking a social history, and even seemingly innocuous questions about demographics, sometimes can pose significant hurdles to

*Training Institute for Suicide Assessment and Clinical Interviewing (TISA), 1502 Route 123 North, Stoddard, NH 03464. (Website: www.suicideassessment.com) *E-mail address:* sheainte@worldpath.net

0193-953X/07/$ – see front matter
doi:10.1016/j.psc.2007.01.006

engagement. A tricky engagement situation can arise when asking clients about their employment. Mike Cheng, MD, provided the following set of valuable tips.

Tip

After the introduction, many clinicians proceed to ask about identifying and demographic data before starting the chief complaint or taking the history of the presenting problem. Often such inquiries start with questions about living situation and marital status. One area of difficulty is asking about occupation.

For example, the clinician should avoid asking a woman, "Do you work?" because that question may imply that a woman who does not have a "paid" job is not working. By implying that domestic chores and/or child rearing is not work, the clinician inadvertently may denigrate the client on a subtle level.

On the other hand, asking, "Do you have a job?" or "Are you working?" may tend to alienate any client who is not currently employed outside of the home. Therefore some interviewers tactfully ask, "Do you have a job or are you between jobs?" Alternatively, the following question may be the most tactful: "Are you working at the moment?" The addition of the words "at the moment" helps the client to "save face."

In the last analysis, because of all of these complexities, the easiest single question to ask is, "How do you support yourself?" This phrasing allows a variety of responses from the client such as: "I'm on disability," or "I work as a teacher," or "My spouse brings in the money for us." From the start, this simple question can provide surprisingly good insights into the employment situation of the client and even how the client feels about his or her current situation.

Clinical Caveat

The interviewing techniques described above provide a variety of thoughtful ways for helping clients to feel comfortable when sharing job status. Another nice question is to ask, "Do you work outside of the home or in the home?"

INTERVIEWING TIP #2: SEVERAL STRATEGIES FOR UNCOVERING DRUG AND ALCOHOL HISTORIES

Description of the Problem

As clinicians all know, it frequently is challenging to uncover valid information when first working with a person coping with alcoholism or street drug abuse. Unconscious defense mechanisms such as denial and intellectualization, as well as conscious distortions, minimizations, and deceit, can hinder the elucidation of valid data. Bruce Berger, MD, provides some nice questions that can help with this common problem.

Tip

I find the following questions useful, particularly in helping to get a feel for the client's understanding of the extent of his or her substance abuse problem as well as the defenses the client uses to avoid facing the impact of the abuse.

For the sake of simplicity, the following questions are phrased for use with alcoholism, but they are equally useful with drug abuse.

1. When you do have periods when you stop drinking, what actually stops you? Do any of the following ever stop you: lack of money, your own sense of self-control, passing out, physical problems like a seizure or a coma?
2. When you are drinking, what do others say about you? Do they ever say you are funny, mean, stupid, or anything else?
3. In your opinion what are the advantages of your drinking to you personally? What are the disadvantages?

Clinical Caveat

With such questions it is interesting to see what the client comes up with during the open-ended phase of the inquiry. At such points one gets a vivid chance to see defenses, such as denial and rationalization, as well as positive characteristics, such as insight and motivation. The more closed-ended inquiries may help stir up some data that otherwise would not be made available spontaneously by the client and also may help the client look at the consequences in a new light.

Notice how Dr. Berger deftly uses the techniques of motivational interviewing [2] in his two questions appearing in #3. First asking the client how drinking helps him—and accepting these benefits as real—opens the door for the client to be more open subsequently in sharing the problems attached with drinking—and perhaps more readily accepting that they, too, are real.

INTERVIEWING TIP #3: THE ONE-WORD DIFFERENCE WHEN ASKING ABOUT SUBSTANCE ABUSE

Description of the Problem

As shown in the preceding tip, one of the classic dilemmas in clinical interviewing is the problem of minimization and denial when clients describe their substance abuse histories. The first task is to help the client to admit to the use of the substance in the first place. The second task is to uncover the amount of use. Kevin Rice, LCSW, addresses the first task in the following simple but effective tip.

Tip

When asking about substance abuse, I find that the word "experiment" almost always elicits a more accurate response than the word "use." An inquiry into the possible use or abuse of marijuana would begin, "Have you ever experimented with marijuana?"

Clinical Caveat

Here is a nice example of how changing just one word can have a surprising effect on the power of a question. Language counts. Sometimes the addition of a small phrase can increase the likelihood of uncovering use even further: "Have you ever experimented with marijuana, even once?"

INTERVIEWING TIP #4: HELPING CLIENTS SHARE CHILDHOOD BEHAVIORS SUGGESTIVE OF SOCIOPATHY

Description of the Problem

Uncovering antisocial or sociopathic behaviors can be difficult, for one must strive to collect valid data about shame-producing behaviors while attempting to maintain a strong alliance. One of the spots that can be difficult is inquiring about antisocial childhood behaviors such as fire-setting or animal abuse. The following tip by Terry Willey, MFT, provides a simple but effective way of raising a difficult subject without immediately alienating the client.

Tip

"When kids are young, sometimes they don't understand their actions and may have hurt an animal while playing with it or being rough with it. Have you ever done something like that, even by accident?"

Clinical Caveat

I like this tip because it raises the potential abuse of an animal in such a way that the client can hint or talk about the incident without an immediately powerful shame-producing admission. Once the topic is broached, the clinician can use skillful questioning to uncover the extent of the abuse and the presence of sadistic pleasure or other evidence of cruelty.

Other antisocial childhood behaviors can be raised in a similar fashion with questions such as, "Little kids are often fascinated by fire and don't really understand its potential dangers. Because of this fact, they sometimes play with fire, or accidentally start fires. Did this ever happen to you?"

INTERVIEWING TIP #5: RAISING THE TOPIC OF PHYSICAL FIGHTING

Description of the Problem

In an initial interview it also can be difficult to raise potentially shame- or guilt-producing topics with which persons have been involved as adults, such as physical fighting, in a gentle and nonconfrontational fashion. Mustafa Soomro, MD, proposes a nice method of raising such topics smoothly.

Tip

I find that if I want to approach the topic of physical fighting unobtrusively, it sometimes is useful to start by raising the topic in such a way that it does not necessarily suggest that the client was involved in the altercation. Once the topic is raised, it is possible to investigate sensitively what role the client played in the violence. In this regard the following question is useful: "Have you ever been in situations where fights occurred and you were affected?"

Using this approach, the clinician can then proceed to flesh out the role of the client in provoking the violence, escalating it, or perhaps merely being a victim of it.

Clinical Caveat

This tip is shrewd and effective. It is very nonthreatening, and it can allow one to uncover all sorts of violence, from street fighting to domestic violence.

It reminds me of another interviewing technique for raising a difficult topic–participation in prostitution–in a way that makes it less shame-producing to discuss by hinting that the prostitution may have been triggered by financial necessity: "You told me earlier that you desperately needed to get money for your kids. Have you ever found that, out of necessity, you turned to stealing or prostitution?" To this nonoffensive inquiry, patients have replied, "You know, I had to turn to prostitution for a couple of months, and I'll tell you one thing, no matter what happens to me, I will never do it again."

INTERVIEWING TIP #6: HELPING THE CLIENT PINPOINT PROBLEMATIC BEHAVIORS OR SITUATIONS

Description of the Problem

Trying to help clients recognize and focus on specific problematic behaviors and times can be difficult, because patients may feel threatened by admitting weaknesses or bad decisions from the past. Caryn Platt Tatelli, AM, LCSW, has developed a nice question that addresses this issue.

Tip

When trying to focus a client on his or her role in the creation of specific problems or difficult situations (such as substance abuse or parenting problems), I find that the following question is often gentle and effective: "If you could turn the clock back to any one point in time, what would you do differently?"

Clinical Caveat

This question is simple and sensitive. It is very different in tone from asking, "What did you do wrong?" because it allows the client to distance from the behavior by taking the lead in supplying some different approaches. A variant of the "miracle question" from solution-focused interviewing (see the article by Michael Cheng in this issue of *Psychiatric Clinics of North America*) also can be effective: "If by some miracle, one thing you did in the past could be turned back, what would you choose it to be?"

INTERVIEWING TIP #7: HELPING PATIENTS WHO HAVE AIDS COPE WITH DEMORALIZATION

Description of the Problem

For patients who have AIDS every day presents a multitude of difficult situations, all of which can lead to demoralization and/or depression. One demoralizing topic that does not always receive the attention it deserves is the huge psychologic hurdle of having to take 14 or 15 pills three or four times a day. Some of these pills are so large that many patients must, literally, gag them down. In addition, for some patients who have AIDS the pills come not to symbolize that they are beating their disease but serve as reminders that they are diseased.

Along these lines, Ed Hamaty, DO, who has specialized in helping patients who have AIDS, offered the following tip in a recent workshop on improving medication interest.

Tip

As the pills become more and more problematic, patients begin to anticipate the unpleasantness of the upcoming pill taking. In essence, they begin to "play a tape" that sounds something like, "Oh God, not this again," or "I can't take this anymore." By working with the patient to come up with a concrete affirmation to say to themselves as they take their medications, this "tape" can be rerecorded into something much more comforting and inspiring.

For example, a patient who has a powerful desire to continue to live to be there for his or her grandchild may repeat the affirmation, "This is for my grandchild."

For a patient who gains a sense of satisfaction from battling back the AIDS virus, the following simple affirmation "Take that!" may function almost like a personal act of releasing defiance.

Each aphorism must be generated by the patient and have unique meaning to the patient. For instance, a patient suffering from intractable pain, may say to the pain as he or she takes his pain medication, "Not today you won't."

Clinical Caveat

These are great tips from Dr. Hamaty, and the range of affirmations is limited only by the imagination and unique qualities of each patient. In essence, the range is essentially limitless.

I am finding these techniques to be very effective with certain patients dealing with psychiatric disorders. For instance, many of my younger patients who have obsessive-compulsive disorder (OCD) find it re-affirming to say something like, "This one is for you, OCD; I'm gonna kick your butt today." Such affirmations externalize the disease so that the patient does not view himself or herself as the problem. They also help the patient to focus attention on his or her ability to control the OCD symptoms, frequently using cognitive behavioral therapy techniques as well.

INTERVIEWING TIP #8: A FAMILY THAT TAKES MEDS TOGETHER STAYS TOGETHER

Description of the Problem

With young patients, the idea that they have been singled out as needing medications can be stigmatizing and hard to process in a healthy manner. The following insightful tip by Rory Sellmer, a fourth-year resident in psychiatry at the University of Calgary, can be quite creative and effective in diminishing this problem.

Tip

I encourage families to take their medications together to normalize the experience. This technique seems to work particularly well with young patients who have psychosis. For example, I might ask, "What would it be like for you if you were to take your antipsychotic medications every night at the same time your Mom is taking her blood pressure medication?"

Parents also can be encouraged to make this a time to check in with symptoms.

Clinical Caveat

Dr. Sellmer first shared this tip with me when I was presenting a workshop in Calgary. It is a delightful way to normalize taking medications, and it can be used frequently, because many parents take some type of medication. It helps the family members view their illnesses, not themselves, as the problem, emphasizing that the family is working together against the illnesses with which they all are coping. In addition, it sometimes may be useful to turn to the adolescent patient and say, "You know, it's also a great time for you to ask your Mom how things are going with her heart problems." This comment further cements the shared reality that "it is us against our illnesses, not us against each other."

CONCLUDING COMMENTS

I hope that you have enjoyed reading these interviewing tips as much as I have enjoyed posting them as the "Interviewing Tip of the Month." I encourage you to visit the Website and see the other tips in the archive. I would also love to receive some tips from you for posting. To me, this type of "Web community and Web sharing" is exactly what the Internet was designed to do. Now let's take a look at some of the tips that our master clinicians have provided us.

References

[1] Shea SC. Training Institute for Suicide Assessment and Clinical Interviewing (TISA). Available at: www.suicideassessment.com. Accessed on March 21, 2007.
[2] Miller W, Rollnick S. Motivational interviewing: preparing people to change addictive behavior. New York: Guilford Press; 1991.

My Favorite Tips for Detecting Malingering and Violence Risk

Phillip J. Resnick, MD

Department of Psychiatry, Case Western Reserve, 11100 Euclid Avenue,
Cleveland, OH 44106, USA

INTERVIEWING TIP #1: DETAILED SYMPTOM INQUIRY

The Problem

A criminal defendant may malinger psychiatric symptoms to avoid criminal responsibility. The ability to detect malingering in a clinical interview is a challenge for even experienced clinicians. One easy symptom to malinger is hallucinations. There are few objective signs that indicate a person is genuinely hearing a voice. For criminal defendants seeking to fake an insanity defense, a common ploy is to allege a hallucinatory command to carry out a crime.

The Solution

The detailed symptom inquiry is a useful technique to unmask the malingerer [1]. The naive malingerer is likely to overstate his or her symptoms based on portrayals of mentally ill persons seen in movies and television. All malingerers are actors portraying a part, but most malingerers do not know the subtle aspects of the phenomenology of psychiatric symptoms. The interviewer should begin with a broad inquiry asking the evaluee to tell all the details he or she can about the onset, course, and evolution of each alleged symptom.

I will illustrate the techniques with the symptom of auditory hallucinations. After the evaluee has described his or her hallucinations fully, inquiry should be made about specific details: for example, whether the voice comes from inside or outside the head; the clarity of the voices; whether the voices converse with each other; whether the voices ever ask questions; the frequency of the voices; whether voices instruct the evaluee to do things, and if so, whether the evaluee feels compelled to obey the command hallucinations.

The subject's answers then can be compared with what is known about genuine auditory hallucinations. For example, 66% to 88% of patients report that their voices come from outside their head; only 7% of auditory hallucinations are vague or inaudible [2]. Genuine auditory hallucinations are intermittent rather than continuous. One third of patients who have hallucinations report

E-mail address: phillip.resnick@cwru.edu

0193-953X/07/$ – see front matter
doi:10.1016/j.psc.2007.01.007

having command hallucinations; the majority of persons who have command hallucinations do not always obey them [3].

One third of patients who have hallucinations report that voices ask them questions. If the evaluee states that he hears questions, he should be asked for examples. Genuine hallucinated questions are not information seeking but tend to be chastising [4]. Thus, genuine voices are likely to say such things as, "Why haven't you written your essay?" rather than, "What time is it?" or "How is the weather?" Questions the interviewer can ask are:

1. Tell me exactly what the voices say.
2. Are the voices continuous, or do they come and go?
3. Do you always feel compelled to carry out the instructions of the voices?

Clinical Caveat

The interviewer should not formulate the question as, "Is the evaluee malingering or genuinely ill?" but instead, whether or not the evaluee has a genuine mental illness, "Is the evaluee malingering specific psychiatric symptoms?" Persons who have experienced true hallucinations may still make up a hallucination to escape criminal responsibility. These malingerers are more difficult to detect because they can rely on their own past genuine hallucinations to answer detailed questions.

INTERVIEWING TIP #2: ENDORSEMENT OF BOGUS SYMPTOMS

The Problem

Although most persons going to clinicians for therapy are honest in describing symptoms, some patients malinger symptoms to gain unjust financial benefits. An easy illness for civil litigants to fake is posttraumatic stress disorder because virtually all of the symptoms are subjective. Another common arena is the evaluation of an alleged psychosis when interviewees are attempting to gain inappropriate eligibility for Social Security Disability.

The Solution

The examiner can ask a suspected malingerer whether he has had rare or improbable symptoms. For example, a patient may be asked whether he has ever believed that automobiles were members of organized religion. Such questions must be asked in the context of other questions exploring psychotic ideas so they do not stand out as unrealistic. Some psychologic tests for malingering apply formal scoring measures to endorsing rare or improbable symptoms. The best-validated of these tests is the Structured Interview of Reported Symptoms [5].

A variation of this technique is to mention to another clinician, within earshot of a suspected malingerer, that a particular symptom is missing that would clinch a psychiatric diagnosis. If the patient then volunteers that symptom, it provides evidence of likely malingering. Questions the interviewer can ask are:

1. When people talk to you, do you see the words they speak spelled out?
2. When you have posttraumatic stress disorder flashbacks do they occur in black and white?
3. Do you find when you are severely depressed that your thoughts speed up?

Clinical Caveat

Evaluees who are mildly retarded or particularly suggestible might endorse rare or improbable symptoms to please the examiner. When unusual symptoms are endorsed, the clinician must integrate this finding with other data before concluding that an individual is malingering.

It sometimes is worthwhile to confront a suspected malingerer with doubts about his or her symptoms. The confrontation should not be done until the examiner has obtained all the information possible from the evaluee. When confronting a suspected malingerer, it is critical to allow the evaluee to save face.

INTERVIEW TIP #3: CONFRONTATION WITH A PARANOID PERSECUTOR

The Problem

Persons who have paranoid psychotic disorders present a special risk of committing severe violence against their "persecutors" in misperceived self-defense. Accurate assessment of homicidal risk in paranoid patients is important to determine if hospitalization is indicated.

The Solution

In addition to inquiring broadly about whether a paranoid person has homicidal ideas, it is effective to confront such individuals with their own specific paranoid persecutor in a hypothetical question. For example, if a patient reports that he is intensely fearful because the Mafia has been following him and trying to kill him, the interviewer might inquire, "Mr. Jones, if you were to see an individual walking toward you in an alley who was dressed like a Mafia hit man, and he had a bulge in his jacket, how would you respond?" One patient might say that he would not do anything because the Mafia has so much power that they could kill him easily if they chose to. A second patient might say that as soon as the "Mafia hit man" came within range, he would take out his .357 magnum and blow his head off. If these patients were asked simply whether they had any thoughts of killing anyone, both might honestly answer no. They have however, different thresholds for killing in misperceived self-defense.

Clinical Caveat

Paranoid psychotic patients are often suspicious of clinicians. Patients who are fearful of being committed may be unwilling to provide truthful answers if they anticipate that such answers will lead to loss of their freedom. Thus, rapport should be established before initiating a question about what the paranoid psychotic patient would do when meeting a persecutor.

STRATEGIC TIPS AND ILLUSTRATIVE DIALOGUE

The clinician in the following reconstructed dialogue has been asked to evaluate a man who killed his mother. The defendant has had four psychiatric hospitalizations and many years of outpatient therapy for chronic undifferentiated schizophrenia and cocaine dependence. This dialogue illustrates both the detailed symptom inquiry and endorsement of bogus symptoms techniques of detecting malingering.

> Clinician: Tell me what led up to the killing of your mother?
> Patient: I was off my medication for 2 months because I couldn't afford it. I started hearing God's voice telling me I should kill my mother.
> Clinician: Tell me about the voice. (detailed symptom inquiry)
> Patient: It was a deep voice continuously from morning until night that said, "Kill your mother because she is a demon." (Genuine voices are intermittent, not continuous.)
> Clinician: Tell me more about the voice. (detailed symptom inquiry)
> Patient: I've heard voices for 20 years. They tell me to do things, and I have to do them.
> Clinician: Have you ever disobeyed the voices?
> Patient: No, I always have to obey them. (unusual response: patients rarely always obey their command hallucinations)
> Clinician: What happens if you don't obey them?
> Patient: They just keep yelling at me until I do what they say.
> Clinician: When is the first time you heard God's voice?
> Patient: I've heard it for 10 years.
> Clinician: Your psychiatric records indicate that you reported no hallucinations since you have been on medication for the last 4 years. Before that, you always reported that your voices were of your dead father.
> Patient: I didn't tell my doctor about the voices lately because I didn't want him to increase my medication.
> Clinician: Do voices ever ask you any questions? (detailed symptom inquiry)
> Patient: Yes they do.
> Clinician: Give me an example.
> Patient: God asked me the number of people who attended my church last Sunday. (atypical hallucinated question)
> Clinician: Has God ever told you that you were going to succeed him as King of the universe? (improbable symptom)
> Patient. Yea. He said that. He said a lot of stuff to me.
> Clinician: Has God ever told you that you should lie on the floor and tremble when he speaks to you? (improbable symptom)
> Patient: Yes. I always lie down when He talks to me.
> Clinician: Did you have any other reason to harm your mother?
> Patient: No, I loved my mother.

> Clinician: Your neighbor told the police that before you stabbed your mother, she heard you arguing with her because she refused to give you $100 from your Social Security check to buy drugs (confrontation of inconsistency).
> Patient: That neighbor is a busybody and a liar.
> Clinician: I know that you have schizophrenia, but the voice of God you are describing now does not conform to what we know about genuine hallucinations. I don't want to write a report to the judge suggesting that you are not being completely honest with me. Could you tell me what else actually led to the death of your mother?
> Patient: Well I didn't really hear the voice of God that day, but my mother had it coming. She's been treating me like a child and stealing my Social Security money.

In this dialogue the patient has the advantage of having experienced genuine hallucinations, so he can answer some detailed questions accurately, but he does endorse bogus symptoms. Furthermore, witness statements and past psychiatric records are inconsistent with the story he is telling. The dialogue also illustrates a face-saving confrontation with the defendant about inconsistencies that result in a confession about faking God's voice.

The next reconstructed interview illustrates the technique of confrontation with a paranoid persecutor.

> Clinician: Tell me what's troubling you.
> Patient: I know that my wife is poisoning me. She and our mail carrier are getting it on and they want me out of the way.
> Clinician: How do you know that this is going on?
> Patient: My food has been tasting funny, so I know she is trying to poison me. The postman also looks at me with murder in his eyes.
> Clinician: Do you have any other evidence?
> Patient: I can just tell by looking at her. She has also had less interest in having sex with me.
> Clinician: Have you taken any steps to try to resolve this?
> Patient: I went to the police, but my wife denied it, and they say I have no real evidence. I started carrying a gun for protection.
> Clinician: What would you do if you were sitting on your porch and the mailman walked up to you and started to take something out of his mailbag?
> Patient: I would have to shoot him in self-defense because I know he and my wife are getting impatient because I am not dying fast enough from the poison.

This dialogue illustrates that the paranoid patient has sought a nonviolent remedy by going to the police to no avail. By learning that the patient would make a pre-emptive strike if the letter carrier approached him directly, the clinician confirms the need to hospitalize the patient.

I have found these three interviewing tips helpful in my treatment practice in addition to forensic evaluations. Although they are useful, no single piece of evidence should cause an interviewer to label someone a malingerer or to conclude that a patient belongs in the hospital.

References

[1] Resnick PJ, Knoll J. Faking it: how to detect malingered psychosis. Current Psychiatry 2005;4: 13–25.
[2] Goodwin DW, Alderson P, Rosenthal R. Clinical significance of hallucinations in psychiatric disorders. A study of ll6 hallucinatory patients. Arch Gen Psychiatry 1971;24:76–80.
[3] Junginger J. Command hallucinations and the prediction of dangerousness. Psychiatr Serv 1995;46:911–4.
[4] Leudar I, Thomas P, McNally D, et al. What voices can do with words: pragmatics of verbal hallucinations. Psychol Med 1997;27:885–98.
[5] Rogers R, Bagby RM, Dickens SE. Structured interview of reported symptoms (SIRS) and professional manual. Odessa (FL): Psychological Assessment Resources; 1992.

My Favorite Tips for Sorting Out Diagnostic Quandaries with Bipolar Disorder and Adult Attention-Deficit Hyperactivity Disorder

Daniel J. Carlat, MD*

Tufts University School of Medicine, Boston, MA, USA

Some diagnoses, such as major depression and obsessive-compulsive disorder, are fairly easy to make. When patients give histories clearly consistent with the *Diagnostic and Statistic Manual of Mental Disorders, fourth edition text revised* (*DSM-IV-TR*) criteria, the diagnostic tasks are easy, and one can move quickly to issues of treatment. As primary care doctors become increasingly comfortable treating basic psychiatric disorders, however, more of psychiatrists' patients are complicated. They do not always fit easily into the neat diagnostic schema that psychiatrists depend on.

This article focuses on two disorders that frequently cause diagnostic quandaries: bipolar disorder and adult attention-deficit hyperactivity disorder (ADHD). But first, here are two suggestions for how to get at the truth of any diagnosis quickly when things are not straightforward:

1. Insist on obtaining past records before the first appointment. True, the patient's last psychiatrist may have gotten it all wrong, but at least the record will give a quick sense of the diagnostic thinking that has trailed this patient and will provide diagnostic clues based on medications that have been prescribed.
2. Ask the patient for his or her diagnosis. This request can be made at the beginning, end, or somewhere in the middle of the interview. I often find it helpful to come right out and ask patients, "Has anyone ever told you what your diagnosis is?" or "So, what do you think your diagnosis (or problem) is?" One patient told me that he once had been diagnosed with trichotillomania—not a diagnosis that I would have embarked upon aggressively without this information.

A reader looking for an extensive exploration of interviewing tips related to all psychiatric disorders, may find my book useful, *The Psychiatric Interview, A Practical Guide, 2nd Edition* [1].

*Corresponding author. *E-mail address*: drcarlat@comcast.net

0193-953X/07/$ – see front matter
doi:10.1016/j.psc.2007.02.008

INTERVIEWING TIP # 1: TAKE NOTHING FOR GRANTED IN BIPOLAR DISORDER

The Problem

Because most patients who have bipolar disorder present initially with depression, the search for mania often involves a fair amount of digging into the history. And because so many of the symptoms of mania are nonspecific, a common pitfall is to conclude falsely that a given symptom is evidence of mania, leading to the overdiagnosis of bipolar disorder.

The Solution

Begin by asking broad screening questions and then focus in on specific *DSM-IV-TR* criteria with questions that can differentiate depressive and anxiety symptoms from true symptoms of mania. The following case illustrates specific examples of such questions.

Case

A 45-year-old married father of three presented with a chief complaint of: "I'm all stressed out." He worked as a construction foreman and said his workers were "driving him crazy." He felt that he had been yelling at his employees excessively. In addition, his wife had been complaining that he was losing his temper with the children too much. One week before the interview, he had returned from a 2-week trip to Asia alone. This was his first trip abroad. He had left without telling his wife, simply buying himself a ticket to Hong Kong.

Initially, the differential diagnosis would include bipolar disorder, anxiety disorders, depressive disorders, and substance abuse. Of these, most clinicians would dwell on the possibility of bipolar disorder, because the patient's impulsive trip to Asia sounds like the behavior of a patient experiencing a manic episode.

A good way to begin the search for mania is to ask a high-yield screening question. Here are some examples I have found useful:

1. Have you ever had a period of time when you felt like your mood and energy were high and your thoughts were going quickly?
2. Did you ever go through a time when you felt too energetic and happy, so that friends commented that you were talking too fast or behaving strangely?
3. Has there ever been a time when you felt just the opposite of depressed, so that for a week or so you felt as if you were on an adrenaline high and could conquer the world?

These questions are good at assessing classic, euphoric mania, but many bipolar patients experience irritability as their primary mood-state during a manic episode. This manifestation is the bane of all interviewers, because irritability is an incredibly nonspecific symptom and is present in depression, anxiety disorders, psychosis, substance abuse, and just about every other entity in the *DSM-IV-TR*.

To understand how to assess manic irritability, it is helpful to recall how manic patients get irritable. Often, the irritability is driven by a sense of impatience with other people's limitations. This impatience, in turn, generally is the result of a combination of grandiosity, excessive energy, and racing thoughts.

Here are a couple of good questions for assessing for the presence of irritable mania:

1. Have you had episodes when you felt that you could think so much more clearly than other people that you became annoyed with them and felt they were getting in your way?
2. Have you had times when you believed that you were superior and more capable than others and got into arguments with people because they were holding you back?

Going back to this patient, here is how the first part of the interview went:

Interviewer: Did you ever go through a time when you felt too energetic and happy, so that friends commented that you were talking too fast or behaving strangely?
Patient: I wouldn't say happy, but I do get revved up.
Interviewer: What do you mean by "revved up"?
Patient: I get a lot of energy, and I can get things done. Mainly at work. But that's when I get stressed out, because there's always too much to do.
Interviewer: Do you enjoy that energy?
Patient: Not really. It's just there; it's my personality. I've always been hyper.

This exchange begins to lead away from mania, because although the patient feels "hyper" and "revved up," he indicates that these are relatively stable personality traits. What about irritable mania?

Interviewer: Earlier, you said that you've been yelling at your coworkers and your family. Why are you yelling at these people so much?
Patient: At work, it's mainly when the guys screw up. It's just normal stuff, they're not bad guys, but when I get overworked, I yell. And when I come home from work, I'm tired, I want some peace and quiet, but my kids are monsters. That's when I yell at them.

The engine of his irritability is not grandiosity and excessive energy, but rather stress and fatigue. So far, the interview is not particularly supportive of bipolar disorder. But what about his impulsive trip to Asia?

Interviewer: How did you decide to go on this trip?
Patient: It was kind of weird, but one Friday, I went to a travel agent and got a round-trip ticket to Hong Kong. That night, I just packed my bags and left.
Interviewer: What was going through your mind?
Patient: That I was fed up with everyone and everything, and I needed to escape.
Interviewer: Did you tell anyone?
Patient: I told my boss I needed a vacation. That's it.
Interviewer: You didn't tell your family?

Patient: Nope. I just left (looks a little embarrassed).

Interviewer: So you just didn't show up at home on a Friday night, leaving your family no idea of your whereabouts?

Patient: No, actually, I told a couple of other friends what I was doing, and I knew they would tell my wife. I didn't want her to be worried. In retrospect, that was pretty irresponsible, I mean I should have talked it over with her myself first. I realize that now.

Interviewer: And what did you do while you were in Asia?

Patient: I was a tourist. I saw the sights. I relaxed. I slept a lot.

Interviewer: Did you spend a lot of money?

Patient: I spent a fair amount on the ticket, but once I was there, I didn't spend much. I stayed in pretty cheap hotels.

Interviewer: Did you do much carousing, drinking, meeting women?

Patient: No, I kept pretty much to myself. And it actually did me good to get away, although I had hell to pay with my wife when I got back!

Again, the story is not very impressive for a manic episode. Although the decision to go to Asia was impulsive and dramatic and fairly screams "mania," with open-minded exploration it seems to be a poorly adaptive response to overwhelming stress. Ultimately, this patient was diagnosed with mild major depression along with an adjustment disorder with anxious and depressed mood.

INTERVIEWING TIP # 2: DISTRACTIBILITY IS NOT ALWAYS ATTENTION-DEFICIT HYPERACTIVITY DISORDER

The Problem

Increasing numbers of people are presenting with the symptom of distractibility and requesting an evaluation for ADHD. Unfortunately, distractibility is a particularly nonspecific symptom that can appear in several other psychiatric disorders.

On one hand spotting undetected ADHD in an adult can be very rewarding. Such patients frequently have extremely low self-esteem and may be viewed as underachievers by both themselves and others. Comorbid depression is common. Treatment can be literally life changing, and, sometimes, life saving if a suicide is prevented.

On the other hand, most people presenting with poor concentration and distractibility do not have adult ADHD. In such instances, an inaccurate diagnosis of ADHD can be quite damaging, because the true underlying diagnosis (eg, major depression, generalized anxiety disorder, substance abuse) will go untreated.

The Solution

Assess the cause of the distractibility carefully.

Case

A 40-year-old woman, who originally had presented with anxiety and depression, came into the office one day and said, "I was talking to my sister this morning, and she said that I'm definitely ADD. She says she just started treatment for it, and it's helping her. What do you think?"

Generally, with such patients the confounding causes of poor concentration and distractibility fall into two common categories: depression and anxiety, and usually both.

The *DSM-IV-TR* demands that the psychiatrist establish that there were symptoms of ADHD in childhood before an adult can be eligible for the diagnosis, but frequently it is hard to establish this retrospective diagnosis reliably. Nonetheless, the patient who reports absolutely no problems with schoolwork or focus as a child is highly unlikely to have ADHD as an adult.

Here are two "fishing" questions that are often answered positively by patients who have true undetected adult ADHD and that may suggest that further ADHD questioning is indicated:

1. When you were a child and adolescent, did you find that it was often a family joke or insider's joke, among your friends, that you were the nutty professor?

People who have severe ADHD (because they are so forgetful, distractible, and late for things) often seem somewhat "zany" to their friends and frequently are the brunt of much ribbing on such matters.

2. When you were going to school, was it common for you to get into trouble for forgetting things like your books, pencils, or homework?

Children who have ADHD usually are "rushing out the door" to school because they are late, and they frequently forget important items at home. Most adults who have ADHD will recall such painful moments of forgetfulness.

Patients, who present as in the case history given previously, however, are often hard to diagnose because their childhood reporting is vague. Most people who had trouble with school did not have ADHD. Moreover, they may even have had some behavioral problems—once again not caused by ADHD. Such self-diagnosed patients, when asked if they were ever treated with stimulants, often say "no" but follow with a quick addendum, "But they didn't give out much Ritalin in those days."

I have found in these cases that the most efficient approach in ruling out ADHD is to start by focusing on depressive and anxiety symptoms. Once those symptoms are fleshed out, one can ask questions such as:

1. When you're feeling good, not anxious or depressed, do you still have significant problems with focus and concentration?
2. When your anxiety goes away, are you able to sit down for an hour and enjoy a book?

Patients who report that their concentration normalizes when their emotional state improves generally do not have ADHD.

It also is helpful to ask patients why they cannot concentrate. Those who have ADHD often respond with, "I don't know why, I just know that I can't focus on any one thing without making a real effort." In contrast, patients who have distractibility secondary to another diagnosis often respond with something like, "Once I start thinking about all my problems, I can't focus on what I'm trying to do."

Some frustrated clinicians just throw up their hands and use a stimulant trial as a form of diagnostic testing. I believe this tactic is not a good idea, partly because even normal people report doing better on stimulants, and also because patients who have primary anxiety may worsen, and even develop paranoia, when taking stimulants.

Ultimately, each patient who enters the psychiatrist's office is unique and difficult to diagnose in his or her own way. The best tip for diagnosing difficult-to-diagnose patients is to listen carefully, take time, and avoid prematurely assuming that one has nailed the correct diagnosis. If we interview with these points in mind, our patients will feel understood, know that we care, and, undoubtedly respond more positively to whatever treatment recommendations we ultimately offer.

Reference

[1] Carlat DJ. The psychiatric interview: a practical guide. 2nd edition. New York: Lippincott Williams & Wilkins; 2004.

My Favorite Tips for Exploring Difficult Topics Such as Delusions and Substance Abuse

David J. Robinson, MD, FRCPC, FAPA[a,b]

[a]Department of Psychiatry, London Health Sciences Center – South Street Hospital, 375 South Street, London, Ontario, Canada N6A 4G5
[b]University of Western Ontario, London, Ontario, Canada

INTERVIEWING TIP #1: GREASING THE WHEELS FOR EXPLORING DELUSIONS

The Problem

It can at times be difficult for patients to discuss their delusional thoughts freely. The reasons for their hesitancy are usually understandable: fear of being viewed as being seriously mentally ill, fear of being hospitalized, or difficulty discussing an emotionally painful situation [1]. At other times, reasons for concealing delusional ideas are illogical or tied to a psychotic thought process, such as auditory command hallucinations that might be telling a patient not to speak with the clinician. Sometimes the patient may even think that the clinician actually is part of a plot or a conspiracy.

The Solution

When patients mention something that could be of a delusional nature, respond with curiosity. An interested, conversational manner helps to elicit detailed information because patients who harbor delusions are generally so immersed in them that the delusions occupy the majority of their thoughts. Your approach is threefold: (1) to grease the wheels so that the patient feels comfortable sharing information, (2) to uncover the extent and logic of the delusional material; and (3) to determine the degree to which the delusion has become entrenched in the patient's thoughts (ie, determine how much insight is preserved or how much distance the patient has from the delusion). Examples include:

1. I'm interested in what you just said; please tell me more. (greasing the wheels)
2. How did this all start? (greasing the wheels)
3. What has happened so far? (uncovering the extent and logic)
4. Why would someone want to do this to you? (uncovering the extent and logic)

E-mail address: dave.robinson@ody.ca

0193-953X/07/$ – see front matter
doi:10.1016/j.psc.2007.01.008

5. How do you know that this is the situation? (determining distance)
6. How do you account for what has taken place? (determining distance)

Clinical Caveat

Regardless of an interviewer's skill, delusional thoughts cannot always be elicited. Patients who have some awareness that others do not share their ideas (preserved insight) or who have been hospitalized previously because they discussed their delusions may choose to conceal their thoughts.

Remember also that if paranoid delusions are present, you must find out if the patient has any thoughts of hurting someone. Questions such as "Do you feel a need to protect yourself against [person in question]?" and "Have you felt a need to possibly take action against [person in question] or harm [person in question]?" are essential avenues to pursue.

Illustrative Dialogue

Clinician: Some people find that, when they experience [insert appropriate symptom, such as depression or anxiety, based on the patient's story so far], their thinking patterns become different. Has this ever happened to you?

Patient: I feel like I can't really think straight and solve everyday problems like I used to, if that's what you mean.

Clinician: Do you have thoughts that you focus on a lot of the time and feel strongly about? (looking for overvalued ideas or delusions)

Patient: I don't understand what you mean.

Clinician: I am asking about ideas that you have that perhaps those around you don't share or agree with, but you know to be true and are puzzled why others may not seem to be convinced and might even argue with you about them.

Patient: I have an infestation with a parasite and asked my family doctor to help me out. Initially she tried, but then seemed to give up and I couldn't understand why, so I've spent a lot of time looking for a nonprescription treatment.

Clinician: That's interesting. How did this start? (greasing the wheels)

Patient: I stepped on a nail about 3 months ago and got an infection. As part of the treatment, I had to soak my foot a couple of times a day. On one occasion, a spider fell into the tub, and you know how dirty those things are. Well, before I could get it out, the water got infected with parasites that the spider was carrying.

Clinician: What happened after that? (uncovering the extent and logic)

Patient: Well, the parasites got into my foot because of the wound and then immediately spread throughout my body causing a variety of physical problems. I haven't been well since that very moment.

Clinician: How do you know that this is the cause of your physical problems? (determining distance)

Patient: Internet research. But before I continue, I need to ask you something?

Clinician: What's that?

Patient: Do you believe me?

INTERVIEWING TIP #2: HANDLING THE QUESTION "DO YOU BELIEVE ME?" WITH A DELUSIONAL PATIENT

The Problem

A major concern of many patients when first sharing a delusion, as in an emergency room setting, is that they will be viewed as being seriously mentally ill. This fear is a natural one for a person experiencing a delusion and to some degree may indicate that the patient has some distance from the delusional material. How the clinician handles this delicate moment may prove to be pivotal to the relationship and determine how much more material the patient will be willing to share. Clinicians do not want to be deceptive, but they need to develop enough of an alliance with patients to hear more about their thoughts.

The Solution

In such situations, you should continue to empathize actively with the patient to preserve rapport and to facilitate the sharing of more information. In addition, you should tactfully avoid being the arbiter of reality and telling the patient whether or not you agree with the patient (or whether or not you think the patient is right) [2]. Examples include statements such as:

1. I'm keeping an open mind.
2. I can't decide without more information.
3. My job is to understand what your views are.
4. The story is an unusual one, so I really want to hear more before making a decision; tell me about . . . [refer patient back into an affectively charged detail from the story].

Clinical Caveat

There is seldom a situation in which you would agree openly with a patient's delusional thoughts (eg, saying something like, "Of course I believe you."). Such false endorsements can undermine a therapeutic alliance and also come back to haunt the clinician later in the interview when the patient asks the clinician to follow through on the endorsement with, "You'll call the police for me, then?"

As with all principles, there are exceptions in which the clinician may need to endorse a delusion temporarily, but these are very rare. Such a situation could arise when the clinician believes that the patient might become violent toward him or her if the clinician does not agree immediately with what the patient is saying.

Illustrative Dialogue

Patient: Do you believe me?

Clinician: I think I can understand why after such an upsetting ordeal that you would wonder if other people believed you. (actively empathizing)

Patient: This has been a real struggle for me. At first there was a lot of concern expressed on my behalf, but as the infestation proved untreatable, people started to voice their disbelief.

Clinician: When did people start becoming less supportive? (actively empathizing)

Patient: After my GP told my family that I didn't actually have any parasites inside of me.

Clinician: What do you think about her saying this to your family?

Patient: It made me very frustrated. I still have the infection, and she not only doesn't believe me, but she can't treat it and now tells my family that it doesn't exist.

Clinician: How is it that this infestation is untreatable for you?

Patient: So you agree that it is untreatable?

Clinician: I don't really know what to think at this point. It is more important that I get a clear understanding of what has happened to you before I come to any conclusions.

Patient: But you have access to all of my records; why can't you make a decision right now?

Clinician: I do have access to your records and have read them, but I prefer to ask you about the situation myself instead of reading someone else's notes. Let's go back to what you believe makes this infestation untreatable.

Patient: Why won't you answer my question?

Clinician: Well, the story is an unusual one, so I really want to hear more before making a decision. Tell me some more about exactly what happened after the spider fell into the bathtub.

INTERVIEWING TIP #3: OBTAINING A MORE ACCURATE SUBSTANCE ABUSE HISTORY

The Problem

Substance use disorders are common in psychiatric populations and have expanded to the point where they may well be considered the rule rather than the exception. Patients often are reluctant to admit to clinicians that they use substances in a nonprescribed fashion, fearing repercussions such as being lectured or having the information included on their medical records. Denial and rationalization, the two most common defenses used by patients who have substance use disorders, only serves to further obfuscate a reliable history.

The Solution

A strategy to elicit a more accurate substance use history starts with waiting until at least half way through the interview to begin this inquiry. This way, the clinician has started to develop some rapport with the patient and, one hopes, is seen as trustworthy with sensitive information. An ideal time to begin taking a substance use history comes after taking the medical history. One can start by asking about legal substance use involving nicotine, caffeine, and alcohol. The use of a structured set of questions (eg, first use, most recent use, amount, effect, and factors perpetuating use) avoids seeming to place added emphasis on illicit or nonprescribed substances. An example is the statement, "Mr. Thompson, many of the patients that I treat did some experimenting with street drugs when they were younger. Often they started with [insert drug here based on patient's history] and then got curious about some others. Because it is vital that I understand your medical health as completely as possible, I'd like to ask what your experience has been with various substances. For starters, did you ever try pot when you were in high school?"

Clinical Caveat

The *Diagnostic and Statistical Manual of Mental Disorders*, 4th edition revised [3] specifies 11 different categories of substances (not including "polysubstance use" or "other"), and it is worthwhile to ask specifically about as many as possible instead of relying on patients to be forthcoming about every experience that they've had. Some patients make a distinction between taking street drugs and misusing prescription medication, viewing the latter as less significant or tacitly sanctioned by their doctors. Also, substances such as inhalants may not be viewed as drugs by some patients. For substances that have parenteral routes of administration, a history of injection becomes vital to help determine the person's risk of being exposed to HIV or a type of hepatitis.

Illustrative Dialogue

Clinician: Mr. Jones, now that we are finishing up your medical history, I'd like to ask about your use of tobacco, alcohol, and caffeine.

Patient: I don't smoke and never did. I drink about five cups of coffee in an average day, but not after dinner because it keeps me from falling asleep. I am a social drinker and usually have wine with dinner on weekends with my friends.

Clinician: Did you ever go through a time where you were struggling with something and found that you were drinking a little more wine to help you cope?

Patient: Yes, I did do that for a while until my wife pointed it out, and I thought that I should ask my doctor about ways to relieve stress. He prescribed a medication for me and told me to stop drinking alcohol.

Clinician: It is very natural for people who are struggling with psychologic stress to try to find something that they can use to help cope better. Did you find that this medication made a difference for you?

Patient: It sure did. It was prescribed to me a few times a day, but I found that when things got really bad, I needed to take it more often than that. It was like a wonder pill for the first few weeks.

Clinician: Sometimes people feel so desperate that they will do just about anything to help themselves feel better. At those times others may not understand or approve, because they just don't know how bad it feels. Did you ever turn to something other than what you have mentioned to help boost your mood?

Patient: I kept hearing about the medicinal effects of marijuana and how it helps some people. I tried that a few times, but it didn't help me.

Clinician: What else did you try? (leading question to help normalize the fact that there may have been others substances used)

Patient: I started to take my son's ADHD medication. It was a real boost for a while, but then I had to get the refills early and knew that I was going to run out of excuses about why the pills weren't lasting him the length of his prescription.

Clinician: Did you ever get to the point where you were taking street drugs or anything else to help change the way you were feeling?

Patient: No, at that point, I realized I needed help and came here.

SUMMARY

I hope that these techniques will prove valuable to you in your daily practice. I also hope that the reader will see ways of generalizing these techniques to other situations in which it may be difficult to engage a patient or to ferret out valid information. I have found that interviewing is endlessly fascinating and that with every patient there is something new to learn.

References

[1] Robinson DJ. Brain calipers: descriptive psychopathology and the psychiatric mental status exam. 2nd edition. Port Huron (MI): Rapid Psychler Press; 2002.

[2] Robinson DJ. Three spheres: a psychiatric interviewing primer. Port Huron (MI): Rapid Psychler Press; 2000.

[3] American Psychiatric Association. Diagnostic and statistical manual of mental disorders. 4th (revision) edition. Washington, DC: American Psychiatric Association; 2000.

My Favorite Tips for Engaging the Difficult Patient on Consultation-Liaison Psychiatry Services

David J. Knesper, MD[a,b,c,*]

[a]Department of Psychiatry, University of Michigan Medical School, Ann Arbor, MI, USA
[b]Hospital and Community Psychiatry Section, University of Michigan Health System, Ann Arbor, MI, USA
[c]Psychosomatic Medicine Program, University of Michigan Health System, Ann Arbor, MI, USA

THE GENERAL PROBLEM OF DISENGAGEMENT AND WORKING WITH THE DIFFICULT PATIENT

Disengagement is the main enemy for the consultation-liaison psychiatrist. Hospital patients referred for psychiatric consultation often are disengaged. Inpatients who occupy a medical-surgical bed self-define their problems as "medical." After all, it was not their idea to be subjected to a psychiatric interview. Against this backdrop, the goal of the first interview is to transform the unwilling, uncooperative, and often difficult and hostile patient into an engaged interview participant. Otherwise, the interview is an unproductive interrogation and an unpleasant power struggle. The three interview-engagement tips or techniques described are among my favorite ways to overcome the impediments to engagement most often associated with difficult patients. Once the difficult patient is engaged, the more typical psychiatric interview can begin.

INTERVIEWING TIP #1: STAYING IN THE RING, MEDIATION, AND DEVELOPING THE THIRD STORY

The Problem

Difficult patients are impossible to interview unless the consultation-liaison psychiatrist overcomes the patient's initial hostility, anger, and sense of entitlement and invalidation. These challenging patients' interpersonal styles are characterized by one or a combination of several defensive character traits. Invalidating, demanding, disruptive, attention-seeking, annoying, and manipulative behaviors are all too common. These patients believe that they are at the mercy of

*Department of Psychiatry, University of Michigan Medical School, UH 9D 9822, Box 0118, 1500 East Medical Center Drive, Ann Arbor, MI 48109-0118. E-mail address: dknesper@umich.edu

0193-953X/07/$ – see front matter
doi:10.1016/j.psc.2007.01.009

an unfriendly professional staff and the likelihood that they may be reacting to feelings of helplessness, fear, and disappointment explain behavior without offering a means to gain cooperation. How do you get started interviewing in this situation? What do you say first?

The Solution

Any medical interview develops out of the clinician–patient relationship. The traditional interview relationship takes one of two forms: active-passive or guidance-cooperation [1]. Expert knowledge and explicit recommendations given to willing and agreeable patients are attributes of both models. Although patients often are told what to do, they seldom protest directly.

Here is a sequence of guidance-cooperation interactions: "I'm here to take you to X-ray." is the hurried and insistent announcement from the transport aide. "I wasn't told I'm having an X-ray today." "All I know is that I've been told to take you to X-ray." "I'm sort of annoyed, but, oh well, let's get going." Perhaps the doctor who ordered the radiograph told the patient in a brief interaction that just did not register, or perhaps the doctor simply forgot to mention this common procedure. Despite being a bit grumpy, most patients get transported to the radiology department without much complaint.

The difficult patient will not go to the radiology department so quietly: "I'm here to take you to X-ray." "Who the hell are you? And which one of my dumb-ass doctors sent you"? "All I know is that I'm supposed to take you to X-ray." "Well, listen to me, Buster! You don't know a damn thing, and I ain't going no place until one of those lazy nurses gets her butt in here and tells me what's going on!" Such raw language and devaluation of professional staff produces strong negative feelings. Typical rejoinders, such as, "You can't speak to people this way," are of no help. Chastising and blaming the difficult patient for misbehavior seems only to make matters worse.

Difficult patients see the situation differently. The problem is, "Nobody told me about going to X-ray." Moreover, the difficult patient feels self-righteous and thinks, "How can I help getting angry when I get no respect?" Now, all of a sudden, the clinician is the one that is supposed to apologize! Predictably, the difficult patient identifies differences that challenge the authority of the clinician, and difficult patients persist until the conflict is resolved in their favor. "Winning" is motivational for difficult patients.

Where to begin? You introduce yourself and the expected reply is, "Leave!" Your first instinct may be some combination of fear and anger. Get past it; don't be intimidated. The first challenge after hearing "Leave" is to stay in the ring and feel comfortable doing so. Your assertive position is made easier by accepting a new role: that of a mediator; it is important to think and act like one.

The key to mediation is found in developing what the Harvard Negotiation Project calls the "third story" [2]. Regarding "going to X-ray," there is the patient's story, the staff's story and the third story. The patient thinks the staff is disrespectful; the staff find the patient rude; the mediator uncovers the third story: both parties could have acted with more courtesy, and both parties would like the atmosphere to change. The third story often is invisible at first. It is only after you understand the other two stories that the third story is developed. Staying in the ring and developing the third story are the most powerful engagement tools you have.

What might be the third story in "going to X-ray"? After peeling away the difficult patient's nasty behaviors, is there a legitimate complaint? I think so. Failure to inform a patient about a medical procedure, however common and painless, is disrespectful. Further, clinical staff is not above passive-aggressive behavior, especially if they have experienced the patient's unpleasantness on previous occasions.

Let's begin: you should picture entering the room, introducing yourself and standing or sitting at a comfortable distance, without crowding the difficult patient. Following the inevitable instruction to "Leave," try your own favorite versions of the following replies:

1. "Before I leave, why don't you and I talk frankly for a moment? [The interviewer can pull up a chair; after all, the interviewer is staying.] You and I both know this is a difficult situation. I'd like to help. I need to understand what you think is going wrong here [patient's story]."
2. "I know you want me to leave [but the interviewer moves a little closer anyway]. That's exactly what I'd like to do, but I'm stuck because many of the staff are afraid of you. Could you help me understand why staff is so fearful? I don't understand it. There must be some good explanation."
3. "Yes, I hear you. I know you don't want to see me, but I cannot leave until I get enough facts to fill out this referral sheet [said while the interviewer waves the sheet]. Maybe we could start by you telling me your experience of the medical care you're getting [a less threatening place to begin]."

Clinical Caveat

Sometimes the patient is so difficult that after you have tried some initial engagement strategies, it is necessary to take time out. "I can see this is not going to work right now; I'll leave and talk to the physician in charge and come back later." Thereafter, the referring physician may need to tell the patient that a psychiatric evaluation is mandatory. Then, one of two things happens: either the physician and the difficult patient have a heart-to-heart talk, with the patient agreeing to behavioral improvement to avoid seeing "a shrink," or the patient agrees reluctantly to the psychiatric consultation. Either way, progress is made.

INTERVIEWING TIP #2: NEGOTIATING, CONCESSION MAKING, AND CONTROL SHARING

The Problem

The problem has not changed. After all, you have just started to develop the third story. What other engagement skills are available?

The Solution

Difficult patients require power sharing, partnering, and mutual participation, and these interview attributes must be the overall goals. To reach these goals, the engagement interview is a process of clinical negotiation. This negotiation is not about who is in charge, or authority, or the clinician's self-image. The interview model based on negotiation is described best by Lazare [3]. Of the several negotiation strategies Lazare recommends, concession making and control sharing are central to engaging the difficult patient. The perceived absence of control is the impediment, and patient empowerment is one means to overcome it.

Clinical personnel dislike any notion of making concessions with the difficult patient. For the consultation-liaison psychiatrist, this situation is an opportunity for liaison work. The fear is that concessions inevitably will undermine clinical authority; staff may believe that "discipline" is what is needed and that it is important not to make exceptions to standard procedures. In this heated atmosphere, it is necessary to do some reframing. There are small concessions, such as agreement and validation; and control sharing may involve simply giving the difficult patient some choices. Making more substantial concessions and giving meaningful control are reframed as "treatment." Generally, difficult patients have a comorbid personality disorder for which specialized therapy is required. Here are some examples of what I mean:

1. "You are absolutely right [concession and validation]. Of course, there needs to be a discussion with you about why you're going to X-ray." (control sharing)
2. "I think I understand how you see the situation and how you feel. Let me tell you your story so I'm sure I have it right." (control sharing)
3. "Yes, it is true that sometimes patients are treated with less respect than any one would like. I can understand why you were annoyed." (concessions and validation)
4. "Yes, you do have a better chemistry with some nurses than with others. I can look into some preferential assignments. This is not what we usually do, but we may be able to make an exception if you agree to be more welcoming ["agree to be more welcoming" is positive; "agree to improve your behavior" is negative.]. (concessions and control sharing)

Clinical Caveat

There is every reason to make some nonstandard changes as part of an overall agreement for improved behavior and cooperation. For example, one nurse or doctor is identified who will spend 30 minutes each morning answering questions and addressing concerns. The patient's room may need to be changed regardless of how inconvenient the change is to the staff. Generally, clinical personnel are willing to make some accommodations if they come to believe they can do a better job as a result, and if they can avoid subjecting themselves to continued unpleasantness. Negotiations make explicit, however, that there are limits to these accommodations and that they are part of an overall agreement. This process is simple contingency management and behavioral therapy. Moreover, if the agreement falls apart, what is given can be taken away easily as part of a contingency-management plan to improve behavior.

INTERVIEWING TIP 3: HONEST LIMIT SETTING AND PLAYING SOFTBALL

The Problem

The difficult patient is demanding and behaving in ways that are unacceptable. Health care services are being compromised. Engagement is impossible unless these issues are addressed during the initial interview.

The Solution

Rather than engaging in tactless confrontation, the interviewer plays "softball," a negotiation strategy Lazare [3] calls "empathic confrontation." The interviewer uses gentle confrontation tactics (ie, "softball"). "Softball" is a clear, assertive, but honest explanation of how and why the interviewer sees things differently and of the limited options available to the difficult patient. The tone is all good-natured.

It is important to be truthful and to establish credibility with the difficult patient. These patients know very well that their behaviors create anger and resentment, and there is no reason to gloss over the real attitudes of medical professionals. Williams and Silk [4] explain that difficult patients sometimes do not know what to do with this honest approach. The basic problem is that the world does not work the way they want, and they are angry as hell about it. Often having been raised in environments ruled by manipulation, exploitation, and hidden messages, difficult patients appreciate straightforwardness. Within reason, validation of their views provides them just enough dignity to motivate both engagement and better behavior. Here are examples of how this approach may be implemented during the initial interview:

1. "Of course you are angry [validation], but when you yell and use raw language, the staff resent having to work with you. They are just human and get upset too."
2. "We cannot work in an unsafe environment. Some of the things you have said, I'm sure you know, frighten people."
3. "I now understand how you see things. [The interviewer could restate the patient's position.] Nevertheless, you can see how busy we are. When we're in a hurry, a standard set of procedures helps us all avoid mistakes."

Clinical Caveat

Unfortunately, many difficult patients are too sick to be transferred to another facility. Unless the psychiatrist lies, what facility will take such a patient? The clinician is stuck with the patient. What can you do if none of these tips work? You must consider other possibilities. Is this patient psychotic? Is this frankly sociopathic and criminal behavior? Criminals have an exquisite insensitivity for the feelings of others. Under any of these circumstances it is important to make sure you are not trying to save the unsalvageable interview. Some interviews are unlikely to improve no matter how skilled the clinician may be. When behaviors are beyond the techniques of negotiation and softball, it may be time for "hard ball." One option is to call the police for support and for a choreographed show of strength. Harassment charges from the staff are unlikely to be ignored.

STRATEGIC TIPS AND ILLUSTRATIVE DIALOGUE

The following dialogue and commentary illustrate one application of the overall strategy. For the duration of the interview, the clinician speaks calmly and is unflappable.

Clinician: "Hi. I'm Dr. Richards. I am a psychiatrist. I'm sure you are happy to see me." (Negotiations might start with a try at paradoxical humor; the interviewer is being approachable.)

Patient: "You're just like all doctors and nurses; you have it all wrong. I am not happy to see you! Who the hell sent you anyway? The last thing I need is a shrink! Leave! Now!"

Clinician: "Alright. I know you were told that I'd be stopping by. You have every right to be angry. Since you've never met me, it's impossible to believe I can be of any help. You're telling me you've been given more trouble than help [validation and small concessions]. Try to tolerate my presence here for just a little while [said while pulling up a chair] so I can explain how I can help. Let's see if we can make the best of this." (The clinician is staying and just introduced developing the third story.)

Patient: (hostile, glaring silence—the patient reacts to having no choice.)

Clinician: "I know you are not happy to see me, but I've been asked to see if there is any way I can make your stay here more pleasant and if I can help you get the best possible health care this hospital can provide." (control-sharing).

Patient: "I'd really rather you leave." (Silence ends; less hostility; deliberate pause)

Clinician: "Frankly, I don't know what is going on [concession, control-sharing], but if it continues you're just not going to get the great care you deserve [softball]. So, tell me what's it been like for you in this hospital." (Curiosity about the patient's story)

Patient: "OK. Now you listen to me! There aren't enough nurses and the few that are here are just plain rude and demeaning. And I see too many doctors! Like is someone in charge here? An army of doctors attack me every morning and treat me like I don't know anything. They don't even want to listen to what I have to say. Gurney-pushers show up unannounced and want to take me to tests no one has told me about. That's the short story."

Clinician: "I cannot tell you how annoying it is to me personally whenever I hear things like this happen. It's true that patients feel often that they are objects on a conveyer belt over which they have no control. I'm sure your feelings are justified." (Concessions; it is too early in the interview to consider the patient's misbehaviors.)

Patient: "OK. So what are you going to do about it, Buster shrink?" (The interviewer must not be intimidated.)

> Clinician: "I'm not sure I know yet. Like you, I'm just one small cog caught in a big health care system. Now, I'm not totally powerless [control-sharing] Tell me what sort of changes might help make your stay better." (control-sharing, developing the third story)
> Patient: "There are too few nurses, and they are all nasty; I need some consistency in nursing care."

Hereafter is a discussion of the third story; this leads to honest limit-setting and softball dialogue that follows.

> Clinician: "I need to be straight with you. I have to be more or less on the side of the nurses. You are going to be here for no more than a week, and then you are going to be gone. But I have to work with these nurses month after month. I simply cannot recreate this medical unit so it runs the way you want it to run."

Softball; or you can try an alternative softball version like this:

> Clinician: "If we cannot find a way to tone this down, I have to tell you that you won't get great care. Every time you tell a nurse to f— off, the word gets around, and nurses will find all sorts of excuses to avoid giving you any extra help. That's just the way the world works, as I'm sure you know. If I were your public relations consultant, I'd recommend we work together to see how we can sort of clean up your act."
> Patient: "Me clean up my act! Hey, I've got the names of some nurses that should be canned; they are just that bad."
> Clinician: "Listen. This is a mess but I'm not going to point fingers at anyone until we [not 'I'] know more [third story]. I've spent the last 30 minutes getting to know you, and I can tell you are doing the best you can under a lot of pressure [concessions]. It isn't any fun to be sick [validation]."
> Clinician: "The professional staff wants to give you the best care they know how. If everyone gives a little and pulls together, this thing is going to work." (control-sharing and the beginnings of a general agreement that is worked out during this and subsequent sessions)

Where is this all heading? The psychiatric fact-finding interview now is possible. Once engagement solidifies, the patient is accessible for a reasoned discussion of behavior. A statement something like the following might open this portion of the interview:

> Clinician: "Before I leave I need to ask you just a few questions so that I can write up that you aren't crazy. [This statement might be said at the outset.] Give me a few minutes to ask you some basic medical-psychiatric questions. You don't need to tell me anything about your personal life." (This is a paradoxical strategy: now the difficult patient is more likely to provide personal information.)

Clinical Caveat

For more information and examples of effective dialogue for difficult patients and difficult conversations, my first recommendation is Brent Williams' and

Kenneth Silk's [4] chapter in *Primary Care Psychiatry*. In *Psychiatric Interviewing: the Art of Understanding* by Shea [5], I especially like the chapter, "The Art of Moving with Resistance." *Managing the Difficult Patient* [6] is another resource. Although not geared to the psychiatric interview, Carter's [7] *Nasty People*, Lerner's [8] *The Dance of Connection*, and Tannen's [9] *I Only Say This Because I Love You* offer excellent suggestions about how to respond to the core features of difficult conversations.

References

[1] Szasz TS, Hollender MH. A contribution to the philosophy of medicine: the basic models of the doctor-patient relationship. AMA Arch Intern Med 1956;97:585–92.
[2] Stone D, Patton B, Heen S. Difficult conversations: how to discuss what matters most. New York: Penguin Books; 1999.
[3] Lazare A. The interview as a clinical negotiation. In: Lipkin M Jr, Putnam SM, Lazare A, editors. The medical interview. New York: Springer; 1995. p. 50–62.
[4] Williams BC, Silk KR. "Difficult" patients. In: Knesper DJ, Riba MB, Schwenk TL, editors. Primary care psychiatry. Philadelphia: WB Saunders; 1997. p. 68–73.
[5] Shea SC. The art of moving with resistance. In: Shea SC. Psychiatric interviewing: the art of understanding. 2nd edition. Philadelphia: WB Saunders; 1998. p. 575–621.
[6] Hooberman RE, Hoberman BM. Managing the difficult patient. Madison (CT): Psychosocial Press; 1998.
[7] Carter J. Nasty people. Chicago: Contemporary Books; 1989.
[8] Lerner H. The dance of connection. New York: HarperCollins; 2001.
[9] Tannen D. I only say this because I love you. New York: Random House; 2001.

My Favorite Tips for Uncovering Sensitive and Taboo Information from Antisocial Behavior to Suicidal Ideation

Shawn Christopher Shea, MD[a,b,*]

[a]Training Institute for Suicide Assessment and Clinical Interviewing (TISA),
1502 Route 123 North, Stoddard, NH 03464, USA
[b]Dartmouth Medical School, Hanover, NH, USA

INTERVIEWING TIP #1: THE BEHAVIORAL INCIDENT

The Problem

All sorts of resistances may predispose a patient to provide distorted information including anxiety, embarrassment, protecting family secrets, unconscious defense mechanisms such as rationalization and denial, and conscious attempts to deceive.

The Solution

The behavioral incident technique was delineated by Pascal [1], who defined behavioral incidents as any question in which the clinician asks about concrete behavioral facts or trains of thought. Pascal notes that to cut through patient distortions, it often is best for clinicians to make their own judgments based on the behavioral details of the story as opposed to the patient's opinions about these behavioral details. He cautions that it is unwise to assume that any person, when asked for an opinion, can objectively describe matters that have strong subjective implications. Instead, Pascal suggests focusing upon the behaviors themselves.

There are two styles of behavioral incident: fact finding and sequencing. Let us look at the high-stakes arena of suicide assessment to see the first style of behavioral incident in action. In fact finding, instead of asking the patient for his opinion (eg, "How close do you think you came to killing yourself?", which can be easily deflected with a quick, "Oh, not that close."), the clinician asks directly about specific behavioral details: "Exactly how many pills did you take?" or "When you placed the gun to your head, did you take the safety off?" Notice how the information gathered by these behavioral incidents may provide more valid data concerning the actual closeness of "pulling the trigger" or "popping the pills" than provided by the question that sought only the patient's opinion.

*Training Institute for Suicide Assessment and Clinical Interviewing (TISA), 1502 Route 123 North, Stoddard, NH 03464 (Website: www.suicideassessment.com). E-mail address: sheainte@worldpath.net

0193-953X/07/$ – see front matter
doi:10.1016/j.psc.2007.02.001

In the second style of behavioral incident–sequencing–the clinician asks the patient to describe what happened next (eg, "What did you do then?") or what thought or feeling came next (eg, "What were you thinking at that moment?") This second style of behavioral incident provides a method for uncovering both behaviors and cognitions in a sequential fashion.

By combining both types of behavioral incidents into a series of questions, the interviewer often can recreate the incident in question by creating a walk-through of the dangerous event, whether it be a suicide attempt or an act of domestic violence. Such sequential walk-throughs are remarkably good at triggering forgotten or repressed material while decreasing patient distortion.

Once again the elicitation of suicidal ideation can serve as a prototype for this strategy. The interviewer poses a series of questions after a patient has reported having thoughts of shooting himself: "Do you have a gun in the house?"; "Have you ever gotten the gun out with the intention of shooting yourself?"; "When did you do this?"; "Where were you sitting when you had the gun out?"; "Did you load the gun?"; "What happened next?"; "How long did you hold the gun there?'; "What thoughts were going through your mind then?"; "Did you take the safety off or load the chamber?"; "What did you do then?"; "What stopped you from pulling the trigger?"

Further examples of fact finding and sequencing behavioral incidents include

1. When you say you "threw a fit," what exactly did you do? (fact finding)
2. Did you put the razor blade up to your wrist? (fact finding)
3. After yelling at you, what did your father do next? (sequencing)

Clinical Caveat

Behavioral incidents are outstanding methods for uncovering hidden information, but they are time consuming. For tasks such as suicide assessment, the increase in validity gained by their use is well worth the time spent. Obviously the clinician must choose when to use behavioral incidents, with a selective emphasis while exploring sensitive areas such as medication nonadherence, domestic violence, sexual abuse, substance use, and suicide.

INTERVIEWING TIP #2: GENTLE ASSUMPTION

The Problem

A plethora of factors can contribute to a given patient's fears of stigmatization. Often a patient may feel that the thoughts or behaviors he or she is experiencing are so weird or bad that "nobody else has ever had such thoughts." One technique for overcoming this obstacle is called "normalization" [2], in which the clinician implies that others have experienced the behavior in question (eg, "Sometimes when people are feeling very depressed, they notice that their interest in sex drops off dramatically. Has this happened to you at all?") Normalization is a great technique, but I want to share another approach–gentle assumption–that I have found to be particulary effective at uncovering highly sensitive material.

The Solution

When using gentle assumption, the clinician, using a gentle tone of voice and nonaccusatory wording, assumes that the suspected behavior is occurring. This gentle assumption metacommunicates the reassuring message to the patient that the clinician has already encountered the behavior in other patients.

The technique was developed by sex researchers, Pomeroy, Flax, and Wheeler [3], who discovered that questions such as, "How frequently do you find yourself masturbating?" were much more likely to yield valid answers than, "Do you masturbate?" If the clinician is concerned that the patient may be "put-off" by the assumption, it can be softened by adding the phrase "if at all," as in, "How often do you find yourself masturbating, if at all?" I have found very few patients to be bothered by the use of gentle assumptions if previous engagement has gone well and the tone of voice used with the gentle assumption is nonjudgmental.

The definition of gentle assumption can be clarified by contrasting this technique with questions that are not examples of gentle assumption. Any question that asks whether or not a client engaged in a given behavior (eg, often beginning with words such as "Have you ever . . .") is by definition not a gentle assumption. For example, when using a gentle assumption to uncover other street drug abuse after having explored the patient's use of marijuana, the clinician would not ask, "Have you ever used any other street drugs?" Instead, the clinician, would matter-of-factly inquire, "What other street drugs have you ever used, even once?" Only the latter type of question demonstrates the technique of gentle assumption.

Other examples of questions that embody gentle assumptions are:

1. What other ways have you thought of killing yourself?
2. What other problems have you had with the law?
3. In the past month how many doses of your medication do you think you may have missed?

Clinical Caveat

No one knows exactly why gentle assumptions work, but they do. Perhaps, as mentioned earlier, they metacommunicate that the clinician is familiar with the area and has seen other people with similar behaviors, indirectly letting the patient feel less odd or deviant. Gentle assumptions also may indicate that, at some level, the clinician may be expecting to hear a positive answer, and it is acceptable to provide one.

Gentle assumptions are powerful examples of leading questions (an attorney on "Law and Order" would be on his feet objecting to each and every one of them). They must be used with care.

More specifically, gentle assumptions should not be used with patients who feel compelled to please the interviewer (eg, a client who has a histrionic or markedly dependent personality disorder) or who might feel intimidated by the interviewer (eg, a child or client with limited intelligence). In such cases gentle assumptions can lead to patients reporting something that is not true, because they feel they are "supposed" to have had the experience or behavior in question. I believe that gentle assumptions are inappropriate with children when exploring potential abuse issues: in such cases gentle assumptions can lead to the production of false memories of abuse.

Before leaving the technique of gentle assumption, it is worth mentioning that sometimes the effectiveness of these validity techniques can be enhanced by linking them into doublets. For instance one could link the normalization technique briefly mentioned earlier with gentle assumption (eg, "Some of my patients tell me it is easy to forget medications, especially when taking them several times a day [normalization]. In the past month how many doses of the medication do you think you may have missed? [gentle assumption]).

INTERVIEWING TIP #3: SYMPTOM AMPLIFICATION
The Problem
Once an interviewer has skillfully uncovered a problematic behavior, a new task arises: determining the extent of the problem. This task brings the interviewer face to face with a most human, but quite problematic, penchant: minimization. Patients often downplay the frequency or degree of disturbing behaviors such as drinking and gambling. One wonders if there is a way to decrease the distortion caused by patients' minimization while maintaining engagement?

The Solution
The use of the technique of symptom amplification, developed by Shea, bypasses the patient's distorting mechanism by setting the upper limits of the quantity in the question at such a high level that, when the patient downplays the amount, the clinician is alerted that there is still a significant problem [2]. For a question to be viewed as symptom amplification the clinician must suggest an actual number.

For instance, when a clinician asks, "How much liquor can you hold in a single night? A pint? A fifth?", and the patient responds, "Oh no, not a fifth. I don't know—maybe a pint," the clinician is made aware that there is a considerable problem despite the patient's minimization. The technique avoids creating a confrontational atmosphere in the interview, even though the client is patently minimizing behavior. Instead, almost in the same way that a martial artist allows the sparring partner's own momentum to drive the opponent to the mat, symptom amplification allows the client to continue to use his or her natural defense mechanisms (in this case minimization) fully while the interviewer still manages to obtain a more accurate snapshot of the extent of the patient's problem.

This technique often is useful in obtaining a more valid history of the extent of violence a perpetrator is displaying (eg, in situations of domestic or predatory violence). If a perpetrator of domestic violence is asked, "How many times have you ever struck your wife?", a typical response, after a few seconds of hemming and hawing, is, "Not often—I don't know—two or three times, maybe." Contrast this information with that obtained from the very same patient when the interviewer uses symptom amplification, asking, "How many times have you ever struck your wife, you know, in any fashion? Thirty times? Forty times? Fifty times?" To this question the same client might state, "Oh my gosh, not 50 times. I don't know. Fifteen times. Ten times. I don't know. It's hard to remember."

It is worth repeating that symptom amplification is used in an effort to determine an actual quantity. It always involves the interviewer suggesting a specific number, set high, with a patient that the interviewer suspects uses minimization as a defense.

Other examples of symptom amplification are

1. How many physical fights have you had in your whole life? Fifty? Eighty? A hundred?
2. How many times have you tripped on acid in your whole life? Twenty-five? Fifty? A hundred times?
3. On the days when your thoughts of suicide were most intense, how much of the day did you spend thinking about killing yourself: 70% of the day, 80%, 90%?

Clinical Caveat

The interviewer must be sure not to set the upper limit at such a high number that it seems absurd or creates the appearance that the interviewer does not know what he or she is talking about. How high the number is set will depend on variables such as the patient's history of past abuse and cultural milieu.

As we saw earlier, it sometimes is useful to combine validity techniques. Sometimes they can be linked into triplets: "Some of my patients tell me it is easy to forget medications, especially when taking them several times a day [normalization]. In the past month how many doses of the medication do you think you might have missed [gentle assumption]—10, 20, 30 [symptom amplification]?"

STRATEGIC TIPS AND ILLUSTRATIVE DIALOGUE

The three techniques discussed here can be woven into a sensitive and smoothly flowing interview. An example of such an interview, reconstructed from an interview with a patient riddled with antisocial traits, shows these techniques at work.

The following dialogue shows how the strategic use of validity techniques makes it difficult for the interviewee to distort the truth through processes such as the parsing of words or relying upon an idiosyncratic interpretation of a word such as "hit." Also, note the power of the behavioral incident to cut away both the patient's distortions and the interviewer's own assumptions and/or projections that also can cast a mist of distortion on the story being told. In this dialogue this phenomenon is most striking when the patient uses the phrase, "I lost it on her."

> Patient: My wife and I haven't really gotten along well in years [pause]. Last weekend we really went at it.
> Clinician: Tell me what happened. (behavioral incident)
> Patient: Well … She just started on me about needing to get a job, that's her big thing now. She wants me to go down to the unemployment office today not

tomorrow. Today. So she starts ragging and yelling and I [pause] I just couldn't take it anymore so I lost it on her.
Clinician: What do you mean "lost it on her"? (behavioral incident)
Patient: I left. Just took off in a fit of rage. I waited till she went out to the kitchen, and I went out the back door, and I didn't come back for 2 days. I didn't call her. I didn't look for a job. I just bagged it all. Screw her.

Many clinicians, including the author, would interpret the phrase "lost it on her" as meaning physical violence. The behavioral incident dismantles this assumption and uncovers a much less disturbing, albeit still pathologic, behavior. Although this assumption would have been off the mark here, the clinician's intuition of violence is appropriate, as is soon shown.

Clinician: Sounds like you two really do go at it. At such moments sometimes people have a hard time controlling their emotions [normalization]. How many times have you found yourself stressed to the point that you may have lost your temper and perhaps hit her [gentle assumption]?
Patient: I've not really done that.
Clinician: What do you mean "not really"? (behavioral incident)
Patient: Well, I've never really ever hit her, not with my fist.
Clinician: Well, have you ever struck her in any way whatsoever? (behavioral incident)
Patient: I slapped her a couple of times.
Clinician: Did you ever slap her hard enough that it caused some bruises? (behavioral incident)
Patient: Not really [pause]. Maybe a black eye once or twice.
Clinician: How many times do you think you have ever hit her? Thirty times? Forty times? (symptom amplification)
Patient: Hell, not that often. Maybe six, seven times.
Clinician: Has she ever had to get stitches or go to the ER? (behavioral incident)
Patient: Oh no, shit no, never.
Clinician: Billy, you told me earlier about all the abuse your father did to you, and it sounded really bad. Sometimes people find that with abusive parents they have to lie to protect themselves [normalization]. Do you know what I mean?
Patient: Hell yea. After he'd had a drunk on, you'd tell the old man whatever he wanted to hear and then you got your ass out of Dodge. And sometimes I had to lie to protect my Mom or my brother.
Clinician: Some people with similar histories of abuse tell me they keep on lying, almost out of habit, even when they are older and sometimes even when they don't want to [normalization]. How often do you find yourself in that situation [gentle assumption]?
Patient [smiles]: Well, Doc, I suppose I lie if I need to.
Clinician: Have you become a pretty good liar over the years?
Patient [bigger smile]: Yea, I guess you could say that.

CONCLUDING COMMENTS
The dialogue in the previous section shows the power of these techniques to uncover domestic violence and antisocial behavior. As I stated earlier, these

techniques are of use in a variety of sensitive areas, from obtaining an accurate history of substance abuse to uncovering medication nonadherence.

Perhaps the most practical and sophisticated use of these techniques is in the elicitation of suicidal ideation and intent as used in the Chronological Assessment of Suicide Events (the CASE approach). Earlier we had seen how the use of the behavioral incident could help the interviewer elicit suicidal ideation more accurately. The CASE approach creates a flexible interview strategy that weaves all of the validity techniques discussed in this article into a method of helping patients share their inner world of suicidal turmoil. The CASE approach is designed to garner a more accurate history of the patient's suicidal ideation over time, including past behaviors, recent planning, and immediate suicidal intent. In the CASE approach, suggestions are made not only for what bits of information my be of use in the clinical formulation of suicide risk, but which of the above validity techniques—and in what sequence—may be best used for eliciting this information in a sensitive and engaging fashion.

For readers interested in learning more details about the CASE approach in clinical practice, see Shea [4–6]. To learn more about its use in the arena of substance abuse treatment, I recommend consulting another article by Shea [7]. Finally, a discussion of how to train clinicians and trainees to use the CASE approach through a method of serial role-playing (macrotraining) can be found online in our Bonus Web Archive at www.psych.theclinics.com by selecting the June 2007 issue, "Clinical Interviewing."

I hope that you have enjoyed this brief introduction to some of the validity techniques currently in the literature. Over the years, I have found them to be of immense value in my clinical work. I think you will enjoy using them and I have no doubt that they will help you to secure a more valid database in many different areas and, quite possibly, save a life some day.

References

[1] Pascal GR. The practica l art of diagnostic interviewing. Homewood (IL): Dow Jones-Irwin; 1983.
[2] Shea SC. Psychiatric interviewing: the art of understanding. 2nd edition. Philadelphia: W.B. Saunders Company; 1998.
[3] Pomeroy WB, Flax CC, Wheeler CC. Taking a sex history: interviewing and recording. New York: Free Press; 1982.
[4] Shea SC. The delicate art of eliciting suicidal ideation. Psychiatr Ann 2004;34:385–400.
[5] Shea SC. The chronological assessment of suicide events: a practical interviewing strategy for eliciting suicidal ideation. J Clin Psychiatry 1998;59(Suppl 20):58–72.
[6] Shea SC. The practical art of suicide assessment: a guide for mental health professionals and substance abuse counselors. New York: John Wiley & Sons, Inc.; 2002.
[7] Shea SC. Practical tips for eliciting suicidal ideation for the substance abuse professional. Counselor: the magazine for addiction professionals. 2001;2(6):14–24.

Our Favorite Tips for "Getting In" with Difficult Patients

Ekkehard Othmer, MD, PhD[a,b,*], J. Philipp Othmer, MD[c], Sieglinde C. Othmer, PhD[b]

[a]Department of Psychiatry, University of Kansas Medical Center, 3901 Rainbow Blvd., Kansas City, KS 66160, USA
[b]Picture Hills Psychiatric Center, 5709 NW 64th Terrace, Kansas City, MO 64151, USA
[c]Department of Psychiatry, VA Medical Center, 4801 East Linwood Blvd., Kansas City, MO 64128, USA

INTERVIEWING TIP # 1: CROSSING OVER TO THE PATIENT'S SIDE OF THE CANYON

The Problem

A patient meets the criteria for a *Diagnostic and Statistical Manual*, edition 4 revised Axis I diagnosis, but refuses treatment, because he or she does not agree that there is a psychiatric disorder present.

The Solution

In such situations it often feels as if the client is standing on the other side of a psychologic canyon from us. To bridge this divide, it may be of value for the clinician first to try joining the client on the client's side of the canyon. This feat can be approached by talking with the client as if the client does not have a psychiatric disorder—walking a mile in the client's shoes—being nonjudgmental while trying to elucidate the patient's main concerns (eg, the practical life problems for which the patient wants help).

With sensitive interviewing, the clinician often can delineate the cause of the client's most pressing distress and propose a solution without ever calling it a "symptom." By focusing on and reducing the client's distress rather than quibbling over the existence of a diagnostic label, clinicians may secure the client's cooperation more readily. We named this interviewing strategy after a song we love, "Canyons Lie Between," that just happens to have been written by our daughter [1].

Case Illustration

Both parents bring Alicia A., a 16-year-old white teenager, to my office. Her long, blue-dyed hair covers her face like a curtain. She has been grounded

*Corresponding author. E-mail address: eothmer@kc.rr.com (E. Othmer).

0193-953X/07/$ – see front matter
doi:10.1016/j.psc.2007.02.007

and/or without privileges for the last 2 years or so because of failing grades and not meeting expectations at home. She states she does not want to be here because she "needs no psychiatrist and no pills." Following a wrist slashing, a brief psychiatric hospitalization did not improve Alicia's mood, although she claims she was never suicidal, and that the cutting was to gain relief. She became disillusioned with her previous outpatient psychiatrist and clearly is not excited about the prospects of working with me.

Patient: I don't want to be here. My parents are making me see you. They try to make me take medications that I don't need.

Interviewer: Your mom says you had good grades up to the sixth grade. Suddenly, your grades went down, and now you have Ds and Fs.

Patient: My grades went down, because I hate school.

Interviewer: So you don't feel depressed like your mom says?

Patient: I told you I hate school.

Interviewer: Your mom also says you have trouble paying attention.

Patient: Why should I pay attention? I hate school.

Interviewer: Dr. P. treated you with medication.

Patient: I didn't want any of those pills. I don't need them.

Interviewer: I agree with you.

Patient [looks up and pushes her hair to the side, glancing at the interviewer with one eye]: So you wouldn't make me take pills?

Interviewer: No.

Patient: Really?

Interviewer: What else do your parents say about your behavior?

Patient: I like Slipnot [a band]. My parents won't let me go to their concert because of my grades. I like Marilyn Manson. My parents hate him. They don't want me to listen to his CD.

Interviewer: What other music do you like?

Patient: I like Rammstein. But they sing in German. I don't understand German.

Interviewer: Well, bring in the CD next time you come to see me. I'll translate a song for you.

Patient: You'll do that? I carry many of my CD's with me. Here is a Rammstein CD.

Interviewer: I'm interested in what you are listening to. When is that Slipnot concert?

Patient: Next Friday at the Beaumont Club.

Interviewer: OK. Is it ok that I talk with your mom?

Patient: You want me to leave?

Interviewer: No. I'm your psychiatrist. Not your mom's. All right then, I'll get your mom in.

Interviewer: Well, Mrs. A., Alicia says she skips medication because she does not need it. She doesn't think that she is depressed. I would like to treat her as if she is right. Let's hold the medication.

Mother: I know she's depressed. She doesn't talk to anybody, goes straight to her room after school and listens only to her music. Dr. P. told us that these are all the signs of depression. But Alicia just shrugs it off.

Interviewer: Depression means having too many bad feelings, like sadness, irritability, and anxiousness, and too little fun. Music is the only joy Alicia has left. I would love for Alicia to have more fun. Punishment can increase negative feelings. It looks like grounding Alicia has not improved her grades. Let's help her have more happy feelings. I suggest you go with her to see Slipnot.

Mother [raises her eyebrows and looks at the psychiatrist with a questioning expression]: But she should earn it, I was told.

Interviewer: You're right. Rewards can help bring about wanted behavior. But in a down mood Alicia may not have enough interest or motivation to earn it. Failure would increase her down feelings.

Mother: Okaaaay?

Patient looks triumphantly at her mother

Interviewer to Alicia: I would like to see you next week. But after the concert, Alicia, I would like you to tell your parents what you like about this kind of music.

At the next meeting, I show Alicia Marilyn Manson's CD "Holy Wood" and I give her the translation of one of Rammstein's songs.

Interviewer: How did you do without any medication?

Patient: I tossed and turned. I couldn't sleep. I woke up early.

Interviewer: Let's fix that. It sucks to be without sleep. It may even make you irritable and cranky.

Patient: Oh, I am already.

Interviewer: Let's get rid of both, the sleeplessness with trazodone and the cranky feelings with Zoloft.

At the next visit Alicia reports:

Patient: I slept and felt better.

Interviewer: Great. If you could reinvent yourself, Alicia, what would you change?

Patient [looking around]: If I could ... hmmm ... you know I would like to be able to stick with things. Finish them.

Interviewer: Let's try something for that. I will give you two different medications. You will take each for 3 days and then tell me which one works better with helping you to stay with things.

Patient: That sounds interesting.

Interviewer: One is called methylphenidate, the other Adderall. I also know a teacher, Mr. G., who makes work fun. I will ask your parents whether they can hire him for you.

At the next visit the patient reported:

Patient: Methylphenidate gave me headaches. Adderall made me tired, but I could pay better attention. Mr. G. really knows how to make me like social studies. He has fun with it himself.

Clinical Caveat

The outcome here was rewarding. The patient went on to have As and Bs with only one C on her next report card. This was quite a turn-around!

Apparently, her previous psychiatrist had correctly elicited Alicia's symptoms and signs and had made the accurate diagnosis of major depression and attention-deficit hyperactivity disorder. He had explained his diagnosis and treatment plan but had not seen that Alicia rejected his "medical model" approach: from her point of view "hating everything" was egosyntonic and "how she felt." In her opinion such feelings/moods and behaviors were not caused by some outside illness.

Joining Alicia by seeing things from her point of view—crossing to her side of the canyon—and treating her without stressing the psychiatric disorder allowed her to feel she was being heard, admit her distress, and accept help. Let me briefly describe, in a stepwise fashion, how I managed to cross the canyon:

1. Her refusal to accept a psychiatric diagnosis: I did not demand that she have "insight" into her problems as potentially being symptoms of disorders and I even stopped her medications (especially because she said she was not taking them anyway, and she reported being nonsuicidal/homicidal). Allowing her to stop the medicines altogether increased her feeling of control and being listened to. Further, if she notices a difference for the worse when the medications are discontinued, she can see for herself the natural consequences of her decisions.

2. Anhedonia: Encouraging fun at a concert, talking about Marilyn Manson, offering a translation of the Rammstein song, and getting a motivational teacher were nonmedical treatments of Alicia's anhedonia, centered around her stated likes and dislikes.

3. Insomnia and irritability: Specifically addressing complaints reported by the clients (such as using trazodone for sleep) builds rapport and, if successful, boosts the stature of the psychiatrist in the client's eyes.

4. Inattention: To increase interest in her school work by finding a motivating teacher fit Alicia's view of her problems. Allowing her to pick her own medication increases her feeling of control, enhancing engagement in treatment and likelihood for compliance.

5. Failing grades: Finding an enthusiastic teacher reduced her anhedonia.

INTERVIEWING TIP #2: CIRCUMVENTING ROADBLOCKS: THE "WHAT IF …" QUESTION

The Problem

Patients, whether in the initial interview or in ongoing therapy, often use everyday language to describe clinically significant psychiatric problems. If the problem remains undiscovered because it is masked by language that typically denotes nonclinical realms, therapeutic roadblocks can arise.

The Solution

First, identify the patient's reported roadblock to social progress (between "better," and where we would like to be, "well"). Second, using the "What if … " question, the interviewer should ask the patient what would happen if the supposed roadblocks were, "as if by magic," removed. This question often can help clarify or discover a missed or unclear underlying cause for a situation.

You then strategically try to see if you, in the interview or in ongoing therapy, can help remove the roadblock (focusing the patient on all the positive things they can do after its removal to see if removal fixes the problem). In the following example, the problem is the patient's being unemployed and not looking for a job; the roadblock is a phobic avoidance of job interviewing rather than a desire to "be disabled" and receive a disability check, as a family member assumes.

Case Illustration

Mr. Mark B. is a 31-year-old PhD student who quit attending classes during relapse of a depression that started after his parents' divorce. He has finished the majority of his course work. A final paper is nearly complete and is all that stands between him and graduation. He is contemplating quitting all together.

He had gone on four job interviews that failed to lead to offers of employment. He became nearly housebound. After his mother left for work, he retreated into her bedroom and watched soap operas most of the day. His father referred him for treatment. At his first visit he reported he was taking sertraline (Zoloft), which had helped him to feel a lot less depressed. Currently, he reported, his mood was more "blah" than depressed. He was pervasively doubtful and felt hopeless regarding most issues. I added Wellbutrin to his treatment. He missed his next appointment.

Several weeks afterward, his father, a certified public accountant, called seeking advice on what to do. He reported that his son continued to refuse to look for work. "He wants to be permanently disabled," his father said. I told the father that, if the patient was willing, they should come in together and bring the mother as well.

At the second visit, Mr. Mark B. was friendly and cooperative, but he presented himself as a failure:

> Interviewer: Mark, how are you doing?
> Patient: Okay, I guess.
> Interviewer: How is your mood?
> Patient: Okay, I guess.
> Interviewer: Is the Wellbutrin helping?
> Patient: Yes.
> Interviewer: So your Dad thinks you should get a job.
> Patient: I'm telling you what I told him. I already tried. It's pointless. No one will hire me. I can't get a job [patient's reported roadblock].
> Father [turning to me]: See? I told you so.
> Interviewer: Now, what if someone hired you, would you go to work? [the "What if . . . " question]
> Patient: No one will hire me. I tried four times. [patient maintains the roadblock]
> Interviewer: I know, it can be hard to get a job, obviously. But, what if you had one, would you go to work? [Clinician persistently, but gently, re-introduces the "What if . . . " question in an effort to identify "where the slip is between cup and lip" in Mark's procuring a job.]
> Patient: Yes.
> Interviewer: Could you do the work and put in a full day?

> Patient: Yes [pause]. But I really don't like interviewing for jobs [hinting at his phobia].
> Interviewer: Well, what if you could volunteer, and wouldn't even need to interview for the job, do you think you could do that? [another example of the "What if . . . " question]
> Interviewer: That would be great. I definitely think I could do that.

Clinical Caveat

I arranged for Mark to be given a volunteer job by a friend of the father. As a volunteer, Mark circumvented the interviewing process. The employer said the commercial value of Mark's work would be $12 to $15 per hour. I called Mark's father and asked him to provide the company the money so that Mark could be paid. Mark was embarrassed by this arrangement. I told Mark that this arrangement saved him from having to beg for every penny from his parents (which had been another point of friction between Mark and his father). After 6 weeks, the father's friend rejected the money from Mark's father and paid Mark directly, impressed by the quality of his work. The company offered to hire Mark, if Mark so desired, which he did.

The "What if. . . " question proved to be invaluable here. Mark completed his thesis and passed his examination. The conflict between Mark and his father over the roadblock—Mark's inability to get a job—had been full of emotion. It had led to anger, fighting, and shouting. Mark's father felt Mark was trying to have a free ride. We helped him to recognize Mark's phobic response. We developed a plan that circumvented the roadblock to Mark's progress. The transformation of the roadblock all began with the strategic use of the "What if . . ." question.

A Second Illustration of the Power of the "What if . . ." Question

Sometimes a patient's self-perceived roadblock can play a role in his or her suicide potential, as we shall soon see in the following case. By using the "What if . . ." question, you can sometimes, with a little luck, help save a life. In this case, the patient, Diane, is a 37-year-old white married woman who reports the symptoms and signs of depression. Her depression started in puberty. She accepts the diagnosis and appreciates my empathy, but her despair is deep. She insists suicide is the only way out of her misery, regardless of what I think or say. Suicide may well be a symptom of her depression, but on a cognitive level, she views suicide as an inviting solution to the meaningless quality of her life.

> Patient: My whole family is crazy and useless. They all abuse drugs. I'm the only one that does not. My marriage sucks. I'm good to nobody. It's time to exit.
> Interviewer: Why?
> Patient: I have no power to help my family.
> Interviewer: How's that?
> Patient: My niece was a crack addict.
> Interviewer: She was?
> Patient: Yes, she was. She was only 23 years old. She's dead now.

Interviewer: What happened?

Patient: I begged her not to go to the 34th Street crack house. She laughed at me and went anyway.

Interviewer: So?

Patient: In the crack house she witnessed the execution of a drug dealer. The executioner murdered her because she was a witness.

Interviewer: How do you know that was the scenario?

Patient: The son killed his own father.

Interviewer: Really?

Patient: Yes, the father had beaten him and thrown him out of the house. The kid was pretty revengeful.

Interviewer: What did you do when you heard this?

Patient: I told my sister I would help her with raising her daughter's two children. But my sister got very depressed. Her younger daughter started to sleep with her to watch out for her.

Interviewer: So how's your sister doing now?

Patient: She overdosed while her own daughter was in bed with her.

Interviewer: What a terrible story!

Patient: That's my family for you.

Interviewer: Why do you want to follow your sister?

Patient: I wanted to adopt my niece's children, but my husband says he'll leave me if I do it. I want to do it anyway, but my lawyer said that as a single parent I cannot adopt two children. [patient's roadblock—possibly a real-world road block]

Interviewer: I see.

Interviewer: What happened to the father of your niece's children?

Patient: He's an addict too. He's in prison.

Interviewer: I feel your distress. You are stuck in a deep hole. [Accepting the patient's existential crisis from her viewpoint is a way of using the first interviewing tip, crossing the canyon.]

Patient: And no way out.

Interviewer: What if you could help your niece's children, would you stick around? [the "What if . . ." question]

Patient: Yes, but I can't, according to the lawyer. [patient maintains roadblock]

Interviewer: I know a single teacher who adopted two kids from Russia. I will get you that lawyer's number. [strategic attempt to circumvent roadblock]

The patient returned for a follow-up appointment.

Patient: Thanks for putting me in touch with this lawyer. The adoption is on its way.

Interviewer: What about your husband?

Patient [shrugging her shoulders]: He's still there. I don't care.

Interviewer: What about your depression?

Patient: I started to take your medicine. I'm still depressed, but those kids need me.

Interviewer: What are your plans to kill yourself?

Patient: I'm still here. Am I not?

Interviewer: Sure

Patient: I started to work out. By the way, I saw you at the YMCA the other day.

Clinical Caveat

The patient measured the value of her life by her power to change some things for the better. Without that power, life appeared worthless to her. I used the "What if . . ." question to help uncover a powerful reason to live—the children of her niece. By subsequently helping remove the roadblock preventing the adoption, I was able to help her choose life over death by suicide. You might be interested to know that the patient currently takes care of her newly adopted children and, in addition, keeps a full-time job. Her husband is still trying to figure out whether he will stay around.

SUMMARY

We never cease to be amazed at the number of methods that exist for transforming roadblocks in the initial interview and in ongoing therapy as well. We have previously described a variety of methods in our books addressing interviewing techniques for use with difficult patients [2–4].

You will also notice that our techniques are similar to those described in an article in this issue by Cheng, regarding solution-focused interviewing, motivational interviewing, and the medication interest model, interview approaches that emphasize a collaborative method for transforming roadblocks by "going with" the client. All these techniques describe methods of creatively "thinking on our feet" during those crucial moments when patients seem to directly oppose us while they wait to see from where we will respond—from an opposing side of the canyon or from their side of the canyon.

References
[1] Othmer JC. Canyons lie between. CD: Oasis Motel track 9. 2006 Available at: www. juliaothmer.com. Accessed February 2006.
[2] Othmer E, Othmer SC. The clinical interview using DSM-IV TR. Vol 1: fundamentals. Washington, DC: American Psychiatric Publishing, Inc.; 2002.
[3] Othmer E, Othmer SC. The clinical interview using DSM-IV TR. Vol 2: the difficult patient. Washington, DC: American Psychiatric Publishing, Inc.; 2002.
[4] Othmer E, Othmer SC, Othmer JP. Psychiatric interview, history, and mental status examination. In: Sadock BJ, Sadock VA, editors. Kaplan & Sadock's comprehensive textbook of psychiatry, Vol. I. 8th edition. Philadelphia: Lippincott Williams & Wilkins; 2005. p. 794–826.

Our Favorite Tips for Interviewing Veterans

James Morrison, MD[a,*], James Boehnlein, MD[a,b]

[a]Department of Psychiatry (UHN 80T), Oregon Health and Science University, 3181 SW Sam Jackson Pk Rd, Portland, OR 97239. Portland, OR, USA
[b]Veterans Administration Northwest Network, Mental Illness Research, Education, and Clinical Center (MIRECC), Portland, OR, USA

INTERVIEWING TIP #1: DIFFERENT AVENUES TO RAPPORT

The Problem

Like so many mental health patients, veterans often come to us with their defenses raised by past experience with caregivers whom they perceive as lacking in understanding. Although health care professionals sometimes find that their own veteran and combat status can afford instant credibility, not all providers have wartime experience to use in developing rapport with their patients. To connect rapidly and effectively with their sometimes suspicious patients, they must find other ways to speed rapport.

The Solution

Of course, the best advice for the clinicians is, just be yourself. Answer questions honestly, admit any deficiencies in your own experience if asked specifically, and in a nondefensive manner point out those experiences you do have that can help the patient accommodate to the treatment relationship. Veterans are just as quick as other patients to identify and resent signs of artifice and condescension. You don't have to know anything about combat, or even very much about the military: in all likelihood, your patient will be delighted to tell you all about it.

In fact, the clinician's willingness to learn from the patient is a powerful builder of rapport. The clinician–patient relationship is inherently lopsided, and allowing the patient to redress some of the imbalance is empowering to the point that it can help the patient feel less suspicious of the clinician and more open and willing to share intimate information. Also, you never know what you will learn about the military service—or any other field of human endeavor—that will help you understand the patient's current situation.

Max, an illustrative case

Max, a 58-year-old Vietnam veteran, presented to the clinic with the chief complaint of nightmares that had been occurring approximately 3 nights per week.

Corresponding author. E-mail address: morrjame@ohsu.edu (J. Morrison).

0193-953X/07/$ – see front matter
doi:10.1016/j.psc.2007.02.002

After many years of virtually no nightmares, they had increased in frequency and intensity dramatically with the onset of the Iraq war. Reading about the deaths of Iraqi civilians had triggered Max's memories of Vietnamese civilian deaths, particularly a family with which he and his unit had become friendly during his year-long tour in 1969 and 1970. These memories in turn had led to nightmares that contained both literal and symbolic images of loss and death. The nightmares and memories had contributed to sadness, irritability, and increased alcohol use over the previous 3 months.

Over the years Max had kept in close contact with several Marine buddies, but they had rarely discussed their Vietnam experiences or subsequent symptoms that they might have had during times of stress. In fact, at the first appointment, Max respectfully told the 40-year-old therapist that he did not want to go into detail about his Vietnam experiences or the content of his nightmares because discussing them made him feel worse. Besides, how could any therapist who was not a veteran and had never seen combat relate to them?

The therapist replied that, despite a lack of veteran status, 10 years of experience working in the Veterans Administration (VA) with veterans of World War II, Korea, and Vietnam had afforded an appreciation of both the unique and universal issues that veterans of all wars face after they return home. Moreover, the therapist mentioned that the confidentiality of the therapeutic relationship might allow the veteran to talk about some sensitive issues or doubts that he had been reluctant to discuss even with his wife or trusted Marine friends. By action rather than by words, in regular sessions over the following several months the therapist communicated to the veteran an ability and willingness to listen, without judgment, to the veteran's painful memories and tearful expressions of loss, mourning, and guilt associated with those left behind in Vietnam.

There is a corollary that even professionals who work for the VA lose sight of from time to time: veterans' experiences may differ, depending upon the era of service. For example, many World War II veterans served for the duration of the war, whereas most Viet Nam draftees returned home after a year. When interviewing veterans, it is always a good idea to ask some open-ended questions [1] to elicit even a brief overview of the patient's wartime experiences and their effect on the individual: "What was your job when you were in combat?"; "How often did you come under fire?"; "How did you deal with your long separation from home and family?"

Clinical Caveat

Like our next tip, this one has virtually no downside. It urges the use of techniques and attitudes that promote a melding of the clinician's desire to gain information with the patient's desire for help.

INTERVIEWING TIP #2: KEEP AN OPEN MIND
The Problem

It happens so often that most clinicians probably have experienced it at one time or another: although the patient's story gradually becomes clearer as time passes and more information comes to light, the clinician—by now invested in a particular theory or favorite treatment—is slow to recognize the emerging picture. Such a blind spot may be especially likely in the face of obvious precipitants such as time spent in combat or a civilian calamity.

The Solution

Throughout history taking, we have found that it is vital not to surrender to complacency but to keep a fully open mind as to the possible causes of a patient's difficulties. Doing so can be a challenge, especially in the face of a patient who has posttraumatic stress disorder with a compelling history of combat trauma.

Burt, an illustrative case

At Burt's first appointment at the mental health clinic, he was queried closely about his combat experiences. He had had "more than a sufficiency of war," as he put it, and the images of explosions, wounds, and dying continued to haunt his dreams. At the end of this evaluation, Burt was assigned to group therapy for posttraumatic stress disorder, and he attended the meetings faithfully for weeks afterwards. Because he continued to have symptoms, the group leader finally asked in private about his marriage. It came out that Burt's wife was complaining about his drinking, as she had done off and on since they were first married, well before he joined the Army. Once his clinicians stumbled onto the fact that something in addition to combat stress might be contributing to Burt's difficulties, it was relatively easy to design a more effective therapy program.

Clinical Caveat

Of course, not all possible causes are equally likely, and one of the clinician's responsibilities is to winnow the list. Doing so too early risks the loss of valuable data; doing so too late can mire the interview in irrelevant material.

The bottom line, and one of our central recommendations is to cast wide the net and consider all diagnostic possibilities [2], even those that initially might seem highly unlikely or even ridiculous. Every once in a while, one of your "unlikely" possibilities will redeem your faith in a broad-ranging differential diagnosis. When interviewing, don't close off any conceivable avenue of inquiry by making assumptions. The same importance attaches to a careful developmental history: childhood loss or trauma may contribute to the frequency and severity of military-related symptoms of posttraumatic stress disorder.

INTERVIEWING TIP #3: DEALING WITH QUESTIONS ABOUT YOUR PERSONAL ISSUES

The Problem

How should you respond when a veteran (or any patient) raises issues or opinions about politics, religion, or other closely held beliefs? This question arises commonly in VA settings, especially with combat veterans, who are often given to expressing their feelings strongly. The answer can pose significant challenges for clinicians. Whereas some patients undoubtedly could handle the give and take of a frank discussion that includes the therapist's own beliefs, it is hard to identify these patients in advance. That's why conventional wisdom prohibits any such discussion in the therapeutic environment.

There are all sorts of ways to deflect such a conversation gambit, some of which only create further problems. Ignoring the question sets you up as someone who either does not listen or does not respond. The simple statement, "I never discuss personal matters," although it might be truthful and is certainly succinct, risks stanching the flow of other, vital information. A seemingly simple and direct response would be to provide the information requested, especially if it is about a belief you and the patient share. These things, however, have a way of leaking out to other patients in the system, and a response that wins you points with one patient might lead later to a more spirited defense than you would like with another, less sympathetic patient. "Why do you ask?" is the tried and true, if hackneyed, response familiar to everyone, but its answer still requires you to craft a response. Reflecting back what the patient has just said ("You seem to feel —") can be annoying, and some patients might think you are mocking them. There must be a better way.

The Solution

Regardless of how provocative (or how far from your own views) the patient seems to be, it is honest to acknowledge the emotion behind the statement: "You really care a lot about this issue"; "I can appreciate how strongly you feel." Then, you can invite further discussion: "How did you come to feel that way?" These responses all have the effect of turning the discussion away from your own preferences and back to the patient's.

If pushed to the point that there is no way out—"Don't you think so, Doc?"—you should respond honestly: "Of course, I have my own feelings about politics, but what I really care about is how you feel. My experience tells me that it is much more important and helpful to focus on the thoughts, needs, and opinions of my patients. Maybe you could tell me what was happening when you first started feeling that way." This forthright statement accomplishes two things: it portrays you as attentive and empathetic, not uncooperative, and it guides the conversation back to the patient's own situation.

Clinical Caveat

It would be counterproductive to proscribe all expressions of personal preference. We generally prefer to be as candid with our patients as possible, which may occasionally include mention of a certain fondness for Savannah, the Sopranos, or salsa verde. It would seem especially pointless to avoid admitting to ideas you have already expressed previously, whether directly to the patient or, perhaps, in a journal article or public lecture. Also, other than religion and politics, the number of topics that you should strictly avoid is small. Even in such contentious topics as electroconvulsive therapy and assisted suicide, your own views can (and should) have a bearing on the counsel you give your patients.

It also is important not to confuse the statement of personal preference with an honest attempt to help clarify the patient's own ideas about matters such as responsibility, guilt, and forgiveness.

STRATEGIC TIPS AND ILLUSTRATIVE EXAMPLES

The explicit subject matter of Tip #3 would seem to render further illustration superfluous. Both Tips #1 and #2 were needed in the following case, however: by focusing on what the interviewer wanted to know about rather than what Amy needed to talk about, the questions from Amy's initial interview (reconstructed long after the fact) conveyed the message that she was right to withhold the meaningful part of her story, which for months she had been afraid to discuss.

Amy, an Illustrative Case

Amy's tour of duty in Iraq had changed her. "All my friends tell me that," she said, wiping away tears. "I guess that's what comes of being a soldier." After that, she grew quiet, volunteering little more about her experiences. The later part of that first interview included this exchange, which illustrates the use of openly admitting a deficiency in knowledge and asking to be taught as a different avenue to rapport:

> Clinician: I can't even imagine a situation where you're at risk for being blown up just driving down a main thoroughfare.
> Amy: Well, after just 3 weeks in the country, I was with several people in my unit when our Humvee hit an IED. My best friend lost the use of her arm, had to be air evac-ed out.
> Clinician: A terrible experience. How did the rest of your patrol handle it?

For several minutes Amy spoke of her tour in Iraq, information about improvised bombs, how she had been taught to scan the roadside for signs that they were there. She also divulged important details about her deepening depression—the crying spells, sleeplessness, feelings of despair. She received a prescription for an antidepressant and was assigned to a group for combat trauma survivors.

In group therapy, Amy mostly just listened. Finally, after weeks of silent attendance, she stopped coming. Within a few days, a senior clinician interviewed her. This exchange includes an example of keeping an open mind as to what else might explain the symptoms:

> Amy: It wasn't helping at all.
> Senior Clinician: What were you feeling?
> Amy: I just couldn't seem to relate to what the others were saying.
> Senior Clinician: Maybe you should tell me what else happened over there.

What came pouring out was a tortured tale of sexual harassment by a few of her fellow soldiers, capped by rape in an empty mess hall by a first sergeant. "He said, if you ever tell about this, your parents are going to get a home visit by two officers in uniform."

References

[1] Morrison J. The first interview. Second edition. New York: Guilford; 2007.
[2] Morrison J. Diagnosis made easier. New York: Guilford; 2007.

Our Favorite Tips for Interviewing Couples and Families

John Sommers-Flanagan, PhD*, Rita Sommers-Flanagan, PhD

Educational Leadership and Counseling, The University of Montana, 724 Eddy Street, Missoula, MT 59812, USA

Individual interviewing differs from couple and family interviewing in one clear and encompassing way: although individual interviewing often includes a focus on or discussion about relationships, couple and family assessment always includes relationships as a primary focus. When interviewing individual patients, the clinician may talk about relationships and relationship dynamics, but when interviewing couples and families, one inevitably observes, experiences, and often is pulled into here-and-now relationship dynamics.

INTERVIEWING TIP #1: RADICAL ACCEPTANCE

The Problem

The problems and beliefs couples and families bring to treatment can be particularly disturbing to clinicians, sometimes causing clinicians to have strong negative emotional reactions to specific couple and family behaviors or statements. These reactions may be reflected in the clinician's nonverbal behaviors or in judgmental statements that, in turn, can reduce patients' openness and cooperation with the interview process.

The Solution

Radical acceptance is a technical modification of Carl Rogers's core attitude of unconditional positive regard. Rogers [1] was comfortable with therapists using techniques as long as these techniques rise up within the therapist in a spontaneous or unplanned way. In keeping with this obvious paradox, we recommend that interviewers use radical acceptance whenever the need for it arises spontaneously. The purpose of radical acceptance is to welcome graciously even the most absurd or offensive patient statements. For example, in response to a potentially disturbing patient statement, one might say, "I'm very glad you brought that [topic] up." Variations of radical acceptance are provided later.

Radical acceptance is especially warranted when patients say something the clinician personally or philosophically opposes. These statements may be

*Corresponding author. E-mail address: john.sf@mso.umt.edu (J. Sommers-Flanagan).

0193-953X/07/$ – see front matter
doi:10.1016/j.psc.2007.02.003

unusual, disagreeable, racist, sexist, or insensitive. Three examples of provocative client statements that might stir negative feelings in the clinician are listed here, followed by illustrations of the radical acceptance technique:

1. Parent [in a parent consultation situation, without children present]: "I believe in discipline. Parents need to be the authority in the home. And yes, that means I believe in giving my kid a swat or two if he (she) gets out of line."
   Clinician: "I'm very glad you brought up the topic of spanking."
2. Husband: "We need to stay together because divorce is against God's law."
   Clinician: "Thank you so much for speaking your mind in here."
3. Parent [speaking to an adolescent in a family therapy situation]: "I can't accept your homosexuality. You have to resist it. I won't tolerate sinful behavior."
   Clinician: "Many parents share views similar to yours but won't say them in here, so I especially appreciate you sharing your beliefs so openly."

Clinical Caveat

Radical acceptance involves actively welcoming any and all comments from couples, parents, and children. To use this technique, the clinician must move beyond feeling threatened, angry, or judgmental about what patients say and embrace whatever comes up.

Radical acceptance, as illustrated in the preceding examples, is more active, directive, and value-laden than traditional person-centered therapy approaches. The goal is for the clinician to communicate his or her personal and professional commitment to openness during the assessment and treatment process. Without such openness, patients may hold underlying beliefs that never get articulated. This perspective relies on the clinician's deep conviction that patients are unlikely to experience insight or be motivated to modify their beliefs unless they expose those beliefs to the light of personal and professional inspection.

Radical acceptance involves letting go of the need to teach the patient a new way. Instead, the interviewer invests in a process that allows unhealthy beliefs to shrink, melt, crumble, or deconstruct with the light and heat of family, couple, or therapist inspection and analysis. For example, in the case of parents who express a need to use corporal punishment, it may be very important for patients to articulate their beliefs in a public/professional setting. Then, after proclaiming such a position and having their rights to have that position affirmed, they may be able to let go of it more completely or use it less often. Similarly, the parent who is unable to accept his or her teenager's homosexuality may need to have painful (and maladaptive) feelings affirmed before moving beyond those feelings and recovering other (more constructive) feelings of love and affection for the child.

When we share the attitude or technique of radical acceptance with clinicians, the first question that arises is typically, "How can I radically accept what the patient says and believes when I also want immediately to help him or her change those beliefs?"

This question gets to the heart of paradox and dialectic in therapy, which Rogers never addressed directly. More recently, however, Linehan [2] and

Hayes and colleagues [3] articulated this paradox and integrated it into their specific therapeutic approaches (ie, dialectal behavior therapy and acceptance and commitment therapy). These approaches emphasize that patient change or progress is stimulated when the patient's emotional condition is completely embraced or accepted. In essence, the interviewer says (and believes), "I accept you as you are, and I am simultaneously committed to helping you change" [4].

In summary, clinicians using radical acceptance welcome and explore all patient statements. Despite this attitude, clinicians using radical acceptance do not endorse all patient statements and beliefs. Instead, after affirming the patient's right to his or her personal beliefs, the clinician may openly question the usefulness or helpfulness of the patient's beliefs or behaviors. The underlying message is that in couple or family therapy clinicians are open to hearing, accepting, and analyzing the utility of anything and everything patients have to say.

INTERVIEWING TIP #2: THE ROMANTIC HISTORY

The Problem

Often, when couples arrive for an initial interview, they are in deep relational conflict and pain. This conflict and pain usually produces negative affect and negative expectations. Consequently, hostile interactions between romantic partners may occur immediately upon the couple's entry into the consulting office and interfere with clinical assessment and treatment outcome.

The Solution

The romantic history—asking how the couple met and fell in love—is a specific interviewing strategy designed to gather information and, at least temporarily, shift couples into a more positive affective state [5]. Shifting couples from a negative to a positive emotional state also can produce more positive exchanges during the initial session. Introducing the romantic history often requires an explanation:

> "All couples have both positive and negative feelings toward each other. Right now, like many couples, you may be feeling more negativity than usual, and you'll certainly get a chance to talk about your negative feelings in here. Right now, however, I'd like to hear a detailed story about how the two of you met, what attracted you to each other, and some pleasant memories from the very beginning of your romantic relationship. Either one of you may go first, but remember, I want to get a feeling for your initial meeting and early romance and so I'll be asking you each a number of follow-up questions."

Clinical Caveat

The purpose of the romantic history is twofold. First, as noted, shifting into a romantic history-taking format can help couples shift into more positive emotional states. Second, research indicates that when couples (or individuals) experience a more positive mood or affect, they can more easily recall other positive experiences and more effectively solve problems [6].

Some individuals resist the romantic history, principally because they want to continue feeling justified in their negative affect or conflict. Additionally, some couples may engage actively in the romantic history but quickly shift back into a negative affect or new or old conflict. Sometimes couples even get into a conflict over their initial romance or share/uncover hidden negative feelings about their early romance. When these situations arise, the following statements may be helpful:

1. "When people are upset or in a bad mood, it can be very hard to remember anything positive, so I'm not sure if you can do this right now." (This statement provides the patient with a small challenge.)
2. "It seems like maybe you don't really want to think of anything positive about your relationship right now, and that's perfectly okay. Whether or not you talk about your romantic history is totally up to you—it's your choice." (This statement affirms the patient's personal control.)

INTERVIEWING TIP #3: TRANSFORMING WISHES INTO GOALS

The Problem

Many couples and families struggle to identify and express their treatment goals. This struggle arises in part because some family members and romantic partners are reluctant therapy participants and have difficulty admitting to problems or believing that treatment will be helpful. Additionally, despite the need for specific goals for insurance and managed care purposes, couple and family therapy patients often, when asked directly, "What are your goals for therapy?", respond with quizzical looks and shoulder shrugs.

The Solution

Early myths, including Aladdin and his magical lamp, speak to the archetypal nature of wishing. Consequently, virtually all patients inherently understand the language of wishes and can identify specific ways in which they might wish their lives were different.

In this technique, the clinician asks the family members to share wishes. The resulting wishes may be transformed easily into treatment goals that are readily agreeable to the family, because they came up with the wishes in the first place. This technique, designed for use when interviewing couples or families, is essentially the same technique as "the miracle question" in solution-focused interviewing described earlier in the Michael Cheng article in this issue of the *Psychiatric Clinics of North America.*

Clinical Caveat

When child or adolescent patients are involved in a family interview, we recommend structuring the wishes into three components [7]. Doing so provides a broader sense of the patient's world and what parts of that world are most troubling:

"If you had three wishes, or if you had a magic lamp like in the movie Aladdin, and you could wish to change something about yourself, your family, or your school, what would you wish to change"?

This question structures goal setting into three areas: self, family, and school. It gives the young patient a chance to identify personal goals in any or all three categories. Depending upon the child and on the parents' influence, there may still be no constructive response. In this case the clinician might try amplifying the question:

> "You don't have any wishes to make your life better? Wow! My life isn't perfect. Maybe I should wish to change places with you. How about your parents? Isn't there a little thing that you might change about them if you could? [pause for answers] How about yourself? Isn't there something small, that you might change about yourself"?

Nervous or shy children/adolescents may continue to resist this questioning process. If so, a chance to pass should be provided.

When using the wishes-into-goals strategy with couples, clinicians must proceed with caution. Specifically, as is generally the rule in couples work, the clinician should avoid giving one partner an opportunity to criticize or suggest that the other partner should make some personal changes:

> "If you had three wishes, but your wishes were restricted to ways in which you might change yourself, ways in which you might improve yourself, what would you wish for? Let me emphasize: these wishes cannot be used to wish for your partner to change in any way. They can only be used to wish for ways in which you might change or improve yourself."

Note that in the preceding example the clinician repeats the limit or rule by which each partner must abide. This repetition or limit setting with couples is strongly recommended because of their tendency to deteriorate quickly into cross-criticism.

Patients who are resistant to treatment typically refuse the opportunity to generate wishes for how their lives might change for the better. They may say things like

1. Everything is fine.
2. I can't think of any wishes.
3. This is stupid.
4. I don't believe in wishes.

The clinician can use the following statement if patients refuse to generate wishes during an interview:

> "That's okay. Sometimes it's hard to think of wishes, or sometimes people don't want to think of any wishes. Let's skip the wishes for now. But, if, at any point, you change your mind and decide you'd like to describe a wish or goal you have for therapy, feel free to speak up."

Additionally, couples often want to wish only for their partner to change. Of course, as noted before, this impulse should be avoided diligently, because usually couples have already been making many statements to each other like, "If only you would listen to me more," or "If you would just accept me for who I am, then we'd both be so much happier." In the end, couples often are relieved to discover their therapist will not let them engage in cross-criticism.

STRATEGIC TIPS AND ILLUSTRATIVE DIALOGUE

The three tips described in this article may be used independently or woven together into a couple or family interview. Obviously, the romantic history is appropriate only within couple counseling interviews. Radical acceptance and wishes into goals may be used during couple, family, or individual interviewing.

The following clinician-patient vignette illustrates the use of radical acceptance, wishes into goals, and the romantic history within the context of a reconstructed single initial couple therapy interview:

> Clinician: I'd like to begin by asking each of you about your goals for therapy.
> Husband: I don't have any goals. She drug me here. I think this is totally stupid. I don't believe in counseling.
> Clinician: Well let me thank you for being so open. It's good to hear exactly what you're thinking and feeling about this [radical acceptance]. I'm especially impressed that you've come for this meeting even though you're totally against it. It says something good about your commitment to your marriage [reframing resistance into commitment].
> Husband: That's right. I ain't giving up on this.
> Clinician: That makes me think we should begin at the beginning. I'd like both of you to tell me, in your own words, exactly how you first met, what attracted you to each other, and some pleasant memories from the very beginning of your romantic relationship. Either one of you can go first, but remember, I want to get a feeling for your initial meeting and early romance, and so I'll be asking you each a number of follow-up questions [romantic history].
> Wife: I'd like to start [at this point, both patients describe their romantic history].
> Clinician: Thanks to each of you for telling me about how you got together. Now I'd like to find out more about what you'd like to do to improve your relationship. But first, let's begin with each of you talking about ways you might improve yourselves. If you had three wishes, but your wishes were restricted to ways in which you might improve yourself, what would you wish for? Let me emphasize: these wishes cannot be used to wish for your partner to change in any way. They can be used only to wish for ways in which you might change or improve yourself [wishes into goals].

SUMMARY

We hope the reader has found this brief description of how to use radical acceptance, the romantic history, and wishes into goals interesting and stimulating. In many ways, we find interviewing couples and families to be the most overwhelming and fearsome of all clinical situations. We have found these techniques are very helpful to couples and families and also helpful to clinicians as they cope with their own feelings and reactions as they interview couples and families.

References

[1] Rogers CR. A way of being. Boston: Houghton Mifflin; 1980.

[2] Linehan M. Cognitive behavioral therapy of borderline personality disorder. New York: Guilford Press; 1993.

[3] Hayes SC, Strosahl KD, Wilson KG. Acceptance and commitment therapy: an experiential approach to behavior change. New York: Guilford Press; 1999.

[4] Sommers-Flanagan J, Sommers-Flanagan R. Counseling and psychotherapy theories in context and practice: skills, strategies, and techniques. New York: Wiley; 2004.

[5] Young-Eisendrath P. You're not what I expected: breaking the "he said-she said" cycle. New York: Touchstone; 1993.

[6] Isen AM. Advances in experimental social psychology. In: Berkowitz L, editor, Positive affect, cognitive processes, and social behavior, Vol 20. New York: Academic Press; 1987. p. 203–53.

[7] Sommers-Flanagan J, Sommers-Flanagan R. Tough kids, cool counseling: user-friendly approaches with challenging youth. 2nd edition. Alexandria (VA): American Counseling Association; 2007.

Part III

Training Psychiatric Residents in Clinical Interviewing: State-of-the-Art Strategies for Residency Directors and Interviewing Instructors

Designing Clinical Interviewing Training Courses for Psychiatric Residents: A Practical Primer for Interviewing Mentors

Shawn Christopher Shea, MD*, Ron Green, MD,
Christine Barney, MD, Stephen Cole, PhD,
Graciana Lapetina, MD, Bruce Baker, EdD

Training Institute for Suicide Assessment and Clinical Interviewing (TISA),
1502 Route 123 North, Stoddard, NH 03464, USA

THE EXTENT OF THE CHALLENGE

"The psychiatric expert is presumed, from the cultural definition
of an expert, and from the general rumors and beliefs about
psychiatry, to be quite able to handle a psychiatric interview."
Harry Stack Sullivan, 1954 [1]

Performing a sensitive and thorough initial interview in 50 minutes is one of
the greatest challenges in clinical practice. Teaching a young psychiatric resident how to do so is, arguably, an even greater challenge.

As psychiatric educators, we realize that interviewing is the foundation from
which all psychiatric care unfolds. It demands psychopathological knowledge,
interpersonal skills, and intuitive abilities. Thus, it is a true blending of science,
craft, and art. It also is a dynamic and creative process requiring a somewhat
elusive set of skills that, frankly, as Sullivan wryly alludes in our opening epi-
gram, may not be part and parcel of every psychiatric graduate's practice.

The importance of this set of skills has been highlighted by Langsley and Hollender [2]. Their survey of 482 psychiatric teachers and practitioners revealed
that 99.4% ranked conducting a comprehensive interview as an important re-
quirement for a psychiatrist. This represented the highest ranking of 32 skills
listed in the survey. Seven of the top 10 skills were directly related to interviewing technique, including skills such as the assessment of suicide and homicide
risk, the ability to make accurate diagnoses, and the ability to recognize countertransference problems and other personal idiosyncrasies as they influence interactions with patients. These results were replicated in a follow-up survey [3].

*Corresponding author. Website: www.suicideassessment.com. E-mail address: sheainte@
worldpath.net (S.C. Shea).

0193-953X/07/$ – see front matter
doi:10.1016/j.psc.2007.02.004

Since the time of these surveys, interviewing, if anything, has become even more challenging, for our time constraints have become more rigid under managed care, our paperwork demands more daunting, and the diversity of cultures from which patients arise—requiring an increased flexibility and sophistication in our interviewing styles—has jumped enormously as we experience new waves of immigration. In like fashion, the designing of clinical interviewing training has become more demanding secondary to factors such as the ever-increasing complexity of the field and our decreasing resources in academia. In addition, some internationally trained residents may require an increased amount of attention as they adapt to the cultural nuances of psychiatric practice utilizing a language that may not be the primary language of their country of origin.

As contemporary psychiatric educators (as well as educators in graduate programs in counseling, clinical psychology, psychiatric social work, and psychiatric nursing) we are facing two core challenges with regard to interviewing training. First, programs must be developed that foster the trainee's ability to handle a wide diversity of clinical interviews with flexibility. The range of interview types includes 50-minute initial assessments, diagnostic interviews, emergency room assessments, consultation and liaison evaluations, medical and psychotherapy assessments, medication checks, and other more specialized tasks, such as forensic evaluations or assessments of trauma victims.

To accomplish this goal, programs must be developed that help residents understand a core set of interviewing principles, that they can then generalize to nurture competence in all of the interview formats described above. These core interviewing principles must help the resident to naturally integrate a wide range of interviewing skills such as engagement techniques, recognition of defense mechanisms and dynamic conflicts, techniques for sensitively structuring interviews, approaches for performing a biopsychosocial assessment that includes the exploration of cultural and spiritual themes, and methods of delineating diagnoses according to the *Diagnostic and Statistical Manual*, Fourth Edition, Text Revision (DSM-IV-TR) and the prospective DSM-V. To top it all off, this massive data-gathering task must be performed in such a way that the patient feels that he or she is having a conversation with a caring professional as opposed to "being interviewed by some guy with a clipboard." This is no easy task.

The second major challenge consists of developing interviewing training courses that are individualized to the specific learning needs of the trainee, for residents vary remarkably in the skill base they bring to their training and in the fashions in which they learn best. It is our experience that the effectiveness of educational techniques may vary significantly with each resident. High resident satisfaction with an individualized approach to learning interviewing has been empirically demonstrated [4].

For instance, some residents may require modeling experiences in order to improve, while others may benefit more powerfully from readings or videotape supervision. We believe that longitudinal, individualized training helps residents secure their newly acquired skills more effectively. This is important, as at least one study suggests that interviewing skills can be easily lost over time [5] and that the intensity of the training has a positive impact on interviewing skill acquisition [6].

This article was written to fill a gap in the literature. Despite the enormous amount of material that has appeared over the years regarding clinical interviewing research (the interested reader can see a review of the literature [7] and an annotated bibliography [8] of recommended readings for psychiatric residents and educators regarding clinical interviewing), we have never come across a no-nonsense primer on how to design clinical interviewing programs.

Such a primer would ideally provide core principles that might help a residency director, course director, or interviewing mentor design a practical clinical interviewing course. Moreover, to be effective, the primer should provide principles that can allow each program designer to create a program that fits the specific needs of his or her trainees within the limiting factors (and there always are limiting factors) of his or her specific residency program.

It is our hope that we have created such a primer and that it will prove to be immediately practical for the busy residency director. If successful, hopefully it will also be fun to read, for, in our opinion, interviewing and the training of the next generation of interviewers should always be fun. The article is informal, and by its very nature, it is a reflection of our personal opinions. It is not presented as the "right way" to teach interviewing but merely as a generator of potential solutions and guidelines.

For those readers who already have outstanding interviewing courses in place, it is our hope that a few nuggets can be culled from this article that may enhance them further. We would also love to hear from you and learn from your own experiences and successes. For those readers who are just starting up a course or are trying to improve their current program, hopefully, this article will provide a sound foundation for further design and implementation.

Throughout this article, I am sharing the considerable expertise of my coauthors who have been intimately involved as interviewing mentors at the Dartmouth Interviewing Mentorship Program (DIMP) that has been running successfully at the Dartmouth psychiatric residency for more than 16 years. Put simply, we are sharing our very best tips on interviewing training design culled from the over 60 years of our combined experience as interviewing mentors.

On a more personal note, it has been my privilege to devote more than 25 years to the study and training of psychiatric residents and other mental health professionals in clinical interviewing, as well as founding the Training Institute for Suicide Assessment and Clinical Interviewing (TISA). Having given over 500 workshops on clinical interviewing and interviewing training design in different academic and clinical settings, I have been able to learn, from clinicians and trainers throughout North America, their best design ideas which I will share in the following pages.

I was also fortunate to be the lead designer in two successful interviewing training programs at psychiatric residency programs. The first interviewing program was in the decade of the 1980s at Western Psychiatric Institute and

Clinic (WPIC) at the University of Pittsburgh, Pennsylvania [4,9]. The second was the DIMP mentioned earlier, which we are describing for the first time in this article. In addition to the innovations of these programs, we also intend to share the mistakes made in each program from which we have learned some painful lessons. Hopefully, we can pass on to you the solutions to these problems, so that you don't have to learn them the hard way, as we did.

Our approach in this primer is four-pronged in nature:

1. Delineate the core principles for designing and successfully implementing interviewing training programs
2. Describe the programs at WPIC and DIMP, thus providing the reader with two distinctly different ways of successfully implementing the core principles in settings where there were radically differing resources and limitations
3. Address some potential problem areas in design and how to avoid them
4. Include, as appendices, some key practical educational tools such as a list of educational goals (regarding the acquisition of clinical interviewing skills) and a sample course syllabus

These tools are not presented as "the final word," but merely as springboards for your own creative design purposes.

THE SEVENTEEN "GOLDEN PRINCIPLES" FOR DESIGNING INTERVIEWING TRAINING PROGRAMS

Principle #1: Use Direct Observation and Mentorship

If the reader were to remember only one principle from this article, the following is the most important thing we have to say: to ensure that a resident has learned an interviewing technique, one must directly observe the resident demonstrating the technique. Direct observation (by being present in the room, behind a one-way mirror, or videotape) is essential for a sound interviewing program. Direct observation is optimized when combined with immediate feedback, coaching, and role-playing until the resident "gets it right." We call this process of ongoing observation and corrective coaching "mentorship."

Clinical interviewing is a profoundly complex procedure. One cannot teach a student how to drive a car by giving a lecture or telling the student to read a book. These educational venues can help, but the bottom line is simple—to teach driving, you must watch the student drive. There is no other way. So it is with clinical interviewing–a behavioral task vastly more complex than driving a car.

By way of perspective, in the state of New Hampshire, where Dartmouth is located, student drivers must have a parent watch them drive at least 20 hours (in addition to taking a driver's education course) before even attempting a driving test. How many psychiatric residents have had 20 of their 50-minute outpatient intakes watched in their entirety by a seasoned clinician before graduating? Bottom line–the more direct supervision you can provide, the better.

We have been consistently surprised at how badly a resident may translate what is an excellent interviewing technique they heard in lecture or read about in a book, into a poor interaction when the resident subsequently tried to utilize the technique with a real patient. Perhaps this fact should not be so surprising, for so much of the power of interviewing techniques depends on nonverbal communication and sensitive timing. Nevertheless, there is only one way to know whether interviewers are translating interviewing techniques from the classroom to the interview room successfully: watch them do it.

It has been a welcome development that residency programs recently have introduced "practice oral boards" where the mock board interview is observed. In no way shape or form, is such an exercise—useful as it may be in the context for which it was designed (preparing one for the oral boards)—a replacement for clinical mentorship in which an experienced coach, familiar with the resident's strengths and weaknesses, sits in the room and directly observes the resident doing actual clinical interviews longitudinally over time.

Principle #2: Focus Upon Learning a 50-Minute Intake

We suggest that, when designing an interviewing training program, you focus upon ensuring that a resident, before graduation, can adequately perform a standard 50-minute outpatient initial assessment. Such interviews are, arguably, the most difficult to perform because of the massive database required while developing a powerful alliance with the patient. More importantly, the interviewing principles used to perform such interviews can be applied easily to other interview tasks. In addition, such an interview may represent the single most common interview that a resident will need to utilize upon graduation being the cornerstone interview required in community mental health work and in private practice.

Principle #3: Model a Complete Initial Interview

Before a trainee can do an initial interview effectively, they must see one done effectively by an experienced clinician from beginning to end. Toward this goal, when beginning a mentoring program with a resident, we often have the mentor perform the very first scheduled interview. It allows the resident to observe a full intake, and it offers, in the post-interview discussion, a chance for the mentor to share things he or she would have done differently if given another chance. This sharing often goes a long way toward "breaking the ice" in supervision. Another option is to have a skilled clinician make a videotape or DVD of a nicely performed outpatient intake, which can then be reviewed by all trainees.

Principle #4: Use Multiple Educational Formats to Provide a Sound Theoretical Framework

A sound theoretical understanding of interviewing goals, techniques, and strategies should be provided either by didactics or book, and we strongly suggest the use of both approaches. Reading can provide a powerful means of consolidating didactic information. It also allows for further exploration of topics that have piqued the student's interest. There are many outstanding major texts, and you can't go wrong with any of the following, which I shall list by alphabetical order of author: Carlat's *The Psychiatric Interview: a Practical Guide* (2nd edition) [10], *The Psychiatric Interview in Clinical Practice* (2nd edition) by MacKinnon et al [11], Morrison's *The First Interview: Revised for DSM-IV* [12], Othmer and Othmer's *The Clinical Interview Using DSM-IV TR* (Vol. 1: *Fundamentals*) [13], Shea's *Psychiatric Interviewing: the Art of Understanding* (2nd edition) [14], and Sommers-Flanagan's *Clinical Interviewing* (3rd edition) [15].

Principle #5: Create an Educational Goals List (EGL)

It is very useful to have a listing of the educational goals, with regard to interviewing skills, which you expect the resident to have addressed by the end of the interviewing course. This educational goals list (EGL) provides the resident with a clear understanding of what is expected and also motivates residents to read more aggressively from the selected textbook, for they can readily see what they know and what they don't know. Equally important, the EGL provides a concrete checklist for mentors to track the development of the trainee's progress, to identify weak areas, and to address these weak areas effectively. Appendix A of this article provides a sample EGL.

Principle #6: Integrate Diverse Mental Health Disciplines

Residents seem to respond enthusiastically to courses that integrate interviewing techniques developed by experts from diverse mental health disciplines. We have found that residents enjoy learning about techniques developed by psychologists, counselors, social workers, and nurses as well as those created by psychiatrists (indeed, some of the most powerful interviewing techniques have come from nonpsychiatric disciplines, such as the "behavioral incident" by Pascal [16] and "motivational interviewing" by Miller and Rollnick [17]). Such training also prepares residents to work effectively in multidisciplinary teams. Nothing helps to cement a sound working relationship with the outpatient psychotherapists in a community mental health center than a psychiatrist who talks glowingly about a technique learned in her or his residency that was designed by a psychologist or counselor.

We recommend describing such techniques in your didactics or choosing a book on clinical interviewing that specifically pulls on multiple disciplines [14]. Note that the presence in the class of different disciplines among the trainees, or the mentors, can significantly enhance this process as well, but is not necessary. In this regard, two of our most popular mentors with psychiatric residents have been clinical psychologists.

Principle #7: Emphasize the Integration of Interviewing Skills

When teaching, it is valuable to emphasize the integration of numerous skills into a single clinical tapestry by modeling engagement techniques, differential diagnoses, and psychodynamic principles in integrated tasks as they appear in actual clinical practice–not as isolated skills. Such integration is enhanced by making sure that the resident knows, while being observed interviewing, the specific interviewing task at hand and is urged to use all available skillsets to do it well. Thus, the trainee may be told to demonstrate a differential diagnosis by the *DSM-IV-TR*, but will be pushed to do so while using specific engagement skills and understanding the psychodynamics needed to help the patient feel comfortable and to increase the likelihood of uncovering valid data.

Principle #8: Place Course in the "Real World"

The course should occur in a setting or clinical rotation in which the importance of the interviewing skills is immediately evident to the resident because they are the exact skills that the resident must use to complete his or her daily work. Thus, the training of an outpatient initial interview should, preferably, be taught on a rotation in which the resident is doing outpatient intakes, not while the resident is solely on an inpatient unit. If at all possible, the observed interviews should be with actual patients that the resident is performing a clinical task and for which the resident will be responsible for the subsequent write-up and triage.

Principle #9: Individualize the Training

We feel that the most effective interviewing training is individualized. In individualized training, the mentor becomes aware of the resident's strengths and weaknesses, and the resident and the mentor have mutually agreed on which interviewing skills are being focused upon in each session of mentoring.

Principle #10: Maximize Learning by Using a Well-defined Supervision Language

It is useful to define the interviewing skills and educational goals with a concise and clarifying supervisory language. The past two decades have seen significant advances in the development of reliable and operational supervisory languages that can greatly enhance the learning of interviewing skills by residents. Naturally, you should choose whatever supervision languages and terms fit best with your own interests and goals.

As an example, I will describe a supervision language–facilics [4,9]–developed years ago that we have found to be quite useful in transforming an almost universal problem with young residents: how do you sensitively uncover the huge database of an initial assessment in 50 minutes, while trying to engage the patient in a conversational mode? Errors range from serious gaps in important data to interviews where rapid-fire questions create a disengaging "Meet the Press" interview style. Of course there are also the one-hour-intakes that run two or more hours in length!

Facilics, a term derived from the Latin root "facilis" meaning ease of movement, is the study of how clinicians gather data and utilize time while trying to engage patients effectively. The language allows the resident to recognize, within his or her own interviewing style, seven different methods (called "gates") of making transitions from topic to topic in an interview. This gating has a lot to do with whether or not a resident's interview feels smooth and conversational to the patient as opposed to stilted and artificial.

Facilic supervision also addresses the interviewer's method of exploring specific data regions with an emphasis on creating a thorough, yet engaging interview style. It further provides the resident with an objective and clarifying look at how he or she uses time constraints effectively or poorly. We have found that facilic principles can be used to better understand, and to more effectively perform, all interview formats from a 50-minute standard intake to a 20-minute emergency room assessment. As an added bonus, an understanding of facilic principles can help the resident to pass the oral boards after graduation.

The supervision system was designed to be easily learned. It also has a set of specific symbols that supervisors use to "map out" the resident's structuring maneuvers as the interview proceeds. This "shorthand" system was designed to clarify educational concepts and to highlight structuring problems and skills, while presenting an immediately understandable visual record of what took place in the interview.

In addition to being useful in coaching the resident immediately after the interview is completed, the graphic system has been useful in videotaped supervision and as a visual springboard for group discussion during class sessions. It also provides a permanent record of the resident's progress over time.

When residents in the WPIC program [4] were asked to rank 12 different educational tools including didactics, role-playing, direct supervision, textbooks, and videotaping, facilic supervision received the most votes as being valuable in learning the art of interviewing. Facilic supervision now is used across mental health disciplines, both nationally and internationally, and has been translated into Spanish, French, and Chinese.

In the DIMP, residents have shown a robust appreciation for the use of facilic supervision. For your convenience, we have provided a guide (and a programed text) to the use of facilic supervision and its schematic shorthand in the electronic version of the article by Shea and Barney, (Facilic Supervision and Schematics: The Art of Training Psychiatric Residents and Other Mental Health Professionals How to Sensitively Structure Clinical Interviews) in this June issue of the *Psychiatric Clinics of North America* in our Web Archive at www.psych.theclinics.com. We hope that you enjoy it and find it useful.

Principle #11: Use the Elicitation of Suicidal Ideation as a Prototypic Interviewing Skill

We believe that all graduates of a psychiatric residency should be able to demonstrate proficiency in the critical art of eliciting suicidal ideation. Indeed, we feel that this skill should be addressed early in the residency, before their oncall duties begin, if possible. In our opinion, a good place to start such training is with the Chronological Assessment of Suicide Events (CASE) Approach, a widely utilized interview strategy that can be taught easily and in which the resident's competency can be tested objectively [14,18–20].

The CASE Approach is a flexible and practical interview strategy for eliciting suicidal ideation and behaviors over four chronological time frames. These four time frames–Presenting, Recent, Past, and Immediate Suicidal Ideation/

Behaviors—are explored using four specific interviewing validity techniques. These four validity techniques: the behavioral incident, gentle assumption, symptom amplification, and denial of the specific, were culled from the pre-existing clinical interviewing literature in the fields of counseling, clinical psychology, and psychiatry.

Because the strategies of the CASE Approach are based on identifiable interviewing techniques, the resident's skills can be easily observed, monitored over time, and objectively tested, ensuring that the resident can effectively elicit suicidal ideation using a reasonable method before graduating the residency.

We recommend the CASE Approach because it has been described extensively in the literature [14,18–20] and has been enthusiastically received among mental health professionals, substance abuse counselors, school counselors, primary care clinicians, and clinicians in the correctional system [21–27]. It is routinely taught as one of the core clinical courses provided at the annual meeting of the American Association of Suicidology (AAS). It is also one of the techniques described in the one day "Assessing and Managing Suicide Risk Course," co-sponsored by the Suicide Prevention Resource Center (SPRC) and the AAS.

From an administrative perspective of a residency director, it is reassuring to know that all one's residents have been trained in a reasonable method of eliciting suicidal ideation, that has extensive face and construct validity, that may hopefully save lives, and that also might significantly decrease the likelihood of malpractice suits. Once again, for your convenience, more information about the CASE Approach, including a method of teaching it called "macrotraining," appears in the electronic version of the article by Shea and Barney, (Macrotraining: A "How-To" Primer for Using Serial Role-Playing to Train Complex Clinical Interviewing Tasks Such as Suicide Assessment) in this June issue of the Psychiatric Clinics of North America in our Web Archive at www.psych.theclinics.com.

Principle #12: Monitor Ongoing Progress

The resident's progress should be monitored in an ongoing and continuous fashion. You may find that a self-monitoring log or journal of what the resident is working on, and their progress to date, can be useful.

Principle #13: Flexibly Utilize Educational Tools

It is valuable to provide access to a range of educational techniques and resources such as a core textbook, supplemental reading list, and various combinations of direct and indirect supervision, always creatively changing educational approaches to the learning needs of the trainee.

Principle #14: Ask for Ongoing Feedback

Ongoing feedback from your residents during the mentorship, including his or her attitudes toward how much they like specific techniques (role-playing, videotaping, etc.) can help you to individually shape the learning experience as it unfolds, maximizing the resident's growth.

Principle #15: Organize a Monthly Mentor's Meeting

If your program utilizes more than one mentor, we feel that it is very important for them to meet routinely as a group, about once a month, for a two hour block. Over the past 16 years, we have found these meetings to be fun and also important for the success of the program. During the mentor meetings, the mentors review the videotapes made by all the trainees, thus offering an opportunity for each of us to spot points for supervision that the trainee's own mentor may have missed. In essence, each trainee gains the input of a handful of different mentors all observing the same tape. It is a uniquely rich training opportunity.

In these sessions, mentors can review the supervision language, ensuring that there is a consistent use of terminology among mentors. We also role-play training techniques with each other. Such role-playing ensures two quality assurance factors: (1) our fidelity to the teaching model and (2) consistency among mentors in the use of the various supervision languages, such as facilics, and in the teaching of interview strategies, such as the CASE Approach.

Also, specific problems with trainees, including resistance to training and problematic attitudes, can be addressed, with creative solutions often resulting. During these meetings, we also make design changes in the course based on resident feedback or changes in resources. Finally, the mentor meetings give a cohesiveness to the group and an identity that helps keep us fresh, so that mentors often stay with the program for years (three DIMP mentors have participated in the program over 15 years).

Principle #16: Update Didactic Classes

Keep an eye on updating didactic classes, for although interviewing techniques and strategies do not change with the ferocious rapidity of psychopharmacological interventions, new ideas do indeed appear. Sometimes entirely new topics emerge in which significant advances have been made with regard to interviewing strategies and techniques. For instance, we have currently added an hour-and-one-half workshop on "How to Talk with Patients About Their Medications" based on new work in this critical, yet often overlooked area. The workshop focuses on the use of specific questions and statements to enhance medication adherence rates while further solidifying the therapeutic alliance [28].

Another interviewing area that has emerged recently which warrants, in our opinion, a class in an interviewing course syllabus, is the topic of cultural diversity. Although attention to this pivotal topic is now required in residency training, we think a specific lecture on interviewing questions and attention to nonverbal differences in culture (from seating arrangement to the role of eye contact) can be valuable.

In addition, we feel that a class devoted to interviewing techniques for sensitively exploring the spiritual beliefs and worldview of patients is important. Josephson and Peteet [29] and Griffith and Griffith [30] have written very practical and informative books on this subject. Be sure to check out Josephson and Peteet's outstanding article on this exact topic in this issue of the *Psychiatric Clinics of North America*.

Another topic that warrants a class, in our opinion, is the rich arena of how to talk with the family members of patients dealing with severe and persistent mental illnesses such as schizophrenia and bipolar disorder, as well as difficult personality processes such as borderline personality disorder. Topics in such a class can describe specific questions and statements that help family members to understand these illnesses, to decrease their stigmatization, to feel comfortable getting their needs met by staff, to ease feelings of guilt and shame, and to learn how to respond appropriately to the symptoms of their loved ones from hallucinations to self-cutting or suicidal behaviors. The article in this issue by Murray-Swank, Dixon, and Stewart is a superb introduction to these interviewing topics.

Principle #17: Use Your Interviewing Course as a Recruitment Tool

Both at WPIC and Dartmouth, we found that our comprehensive interviewing training programs were powerful recruitment tools for attracting high-quality residents. Resident applicants were well aware that interviewing skills were critical to their training and were impressed by the presence of interviewing mentorship, in addition to psychotherapy supervision, at both the WPIC and the Dartmouth programs.

TWO SAMPLE INTERVIEWING TRAINING PROGRAMS: STRENGTHS AND WEAKNESSES

We doubt that an ideal interviewing training program can ever be created. Resources in contemporary residency training are simply far too scarce to do so. Moreover, an "ideal" interviewing training program that cannot be implemented is not ideal; it is foolish. Thus, we are all faced with the tough task of designing the best interviewing training programs that we can with the resources we have available. In some instances, the program that is designed may be fairly minimal, but a well-thought-out minimal program is still much better than no program at all, especially if (1) it sparks the interest of the resident to further improve his or her interviewing skills and (2) provides the theoretical framework from which the resident can do so.

On the bright side, we don't think that most programs must be minimal in nature, nor should they be minimal considering the immense importance of clinical interviewing skills. Armed with a sound theoretical approach to designing interviewing training programs—as we are trying to provide in this primer—we feel that surprisingly robust programs can be developed even with limited resources.

In the following section, we will show two widely differing programs that we feel have been very successful, as indicated by resident satisfaction and longevity of the programs. It is hoped that they will provide models from which the reader can pick and choose bits and pieces to create a viable and lively program in their own psychiatry department.

For the most part, each of the programs implements all the core principles listed above. Naturally, each program implements them with varying degrees of efficacy secondary to limitations on the number of mentors, institutional politics, resident's schedules, and the availability of clinical rotations willing to support the training. Consequently, the strengths and weaknesses of each program will be addressed as well.

We want to emphasize that a high-quality interviewing training program does not have to incorporate all 17 principles described in the previous section. Rather, we are saying that by incorporating as many of the principles as resources allow, you are likely to maximize the benefits of your program and minimize its weaknesses.

Western Psychiatric Institute and Clinic (WPIC) Interviewing Course (1983–1988)

The biggest challenge for this program design—and it was a big one—was that only one faculty member (myself) was available to teach a course on interviewing while trying to provide mentorship to more than 40 residents (slightly more than ten a year). Such a limited teaching force is fairly common, and this program demonstrates some methods that might help you navigate such a challenge.

To begin with, in order to offset the obvious decrease in time that could be devoted to mentoring, this course emphasized the use of didactic material, but I tried to make sure that all the didactic material could be immediately applied to the direct clinical experience and supervision of the residents. Consequently, placement of the course became critical, and I looked for a spot where, even though I could only provide two or three sessions of direct mentoring, the resident might be able to observe interviewing by other experienced faculty and perhaps receive some feedback from them as well.

The training program subsequently was integrated into the three month rotation at the Diagnostic and Evaluation Center (DEC) at WPIC, of which I was the medical director. Residents usually hit this rotation during postgraduate year (PGY) II or PGY III. This unit functioned both as a full intake assessment center and as a psychiatric emergency room. Several times a day while on this rotation, residents were required to conduct two significantly different styles of interview tailored to the clinical task at hand, classic 50-minute intakes and 20- to 30-minute emergency room assessments. After the resident interviewed the patient and presented to a faculty psychiatrist, the patient was also interviewed briefly by the faculty, providing the resident a chance to observe the faculty member's interaction with the patient.

During the rotation, residents attended 17 1.5-hour classes dedicated to interviewing techniques (In Appendix B, a prototype of a class syllabus is provided for your use that has been further expanded and improved upon from my subsequent experience over the years). The first 30 minutes was devoted to lecture. In the second 30 minutes, one of the trainees interviewed a patient from the DEC (or from an inpatient unit if no clinic patient was available) in front of the class with all participants in the same room as the interviewing dyad. In the last 30 minutes, the group discussed the interview and provided constructive feedback (partially compensating for the lack of direct mentorship).

Classes were composed of 6 to 14 mental health trainees including psychiatric residents, clinical psychology interns, psychiatric nurses, social work interns, family practice residents, emergency medicine residents, counseling students, and medical students. This multidisciplinary learning cohort provided a rich arena for personal growth and learning. The lectures and readings (a draft of my eventual textbook, *Psychiatric Interviewing: the Art of Understanding,* which evolved from the lectures themselves) provided a theoretical overview covering the Educational Goals List (EGL), while integrating numerous schools of thought and disciplines including descriptive psychopathology, psychoanalysis, counseling, and clinical psychology.

From an experiential perspective each resident had to observe at least two videotaped intakes from our experienced staff. I only had time to provide direct supervision (mentorship) to the psychiatric residents. Two forms of direct supervision were used. Each resident videotaped an initial intake, which I then reviewed alone first, and then reviewed together with the resident to pick out a few areas for improvement. Subsequently, I sat in and directly observed the resident's entire interview (sometimes demonstrating specific techniques) on two or three occasions.

The strengths of this program are obvious. For a more detailed description, including empiric data on resident satisfaction, the following papers [4,9] will be of value.) In my opinion, the theoretical framework provided by the lectures and the textbook was pivotal to the success of the program. Having this material immediately amplified by watching another trainee's interview, and then discussing it as a group, enhanced both enthusiasm and understanding. It was also hard to beat the rich multidisciplinary milieu, and it was gratifying to see the interdisciplinary walls fall as the course proceeded and genuine cross-discipline respect grew.

Residents also reported benefiting greatly from the review of their videotape, which was completely mapped out using facilic schematics. The majority of residents reported that one of the most powerful learning experiences was the two or three sessions of subsequent direct mentorship with me sitting in the room as the interview proceeded, once again noting the facilics of their interview. Residents strongly urged that the number of direct mentorship sessions be markedly increased. Alas, I could only do 2-3 because of time constraints, which was the most striking deficit of the program, a deficit that in the DIMP would be dramatically addressed.

Dartmouth Interviewing Mentorship (DIMP) Program (1989–2004)

In the Dartmouth interviewing program, we were able to capitalize on all that had been learned at WPIC, but we also had some new limiting factors. Specifically, since I was an adjunct faculty and lived 1.5 hours from the Dartmouth Medical Center, it was not feasible for me to both teach a 17-class course and to attend monthly mentors' meetings. Thus, we had to come up with a different way to approach the didactic teaching component of the program.

From the experiences at WPIC, it was clear, from the empirical resident feedback, that the most popular learning came from direct mentorship. Consequently, we wanted to turn the thrust of our resources towards providing a longitudinal mentorship experience for the residents.

By presenting at Grand Rounds outlining the core principles of designing an ongoing interviewing mentorship program (which included a description of facilic supervision, elements of the CASE Approach, and my experiences at WPIC), we had over 10 faculty who wanted to become interviewing mentors. By the time we were done training the volunteer faculty over the next year we had a solid core of six committed interviewing mentors, for the most part allowing each mentor to work with one resident per year.

To address the absence of an ongoing didactic class, as had been present at WPIC, we decided to emphasize the textbook [14] as the cornerstone of the ongoing didactics, for it comprehensively covered almost all of the material in our EGL as well as introducing the student to facilics, the CASE Approach, and several other interviewing languages that had proved popular at WPIC (eg, the teaching of validity techniques including the behavioral incident, shame attenuation, gentle assumption, symptom amplification, and denial of the specific, as well as a supervision language called the "Degree of Openness Continuum" (DOC) that gave residents an objective awareness of the style of questions they were using.)

In addition, the year-long mentorship, placed into the PGY III year when residents were doing their outpatient clinics, was "kicked-off" with two full-day workshops given 1 week apart. Each day had four workshops of 1.5 hours. Topics covered included

Day 1:

1. The Initial Interview; Traps, Roadblocks, Strategies and Solutions (which included a complete experiential introduction to the facilic system and schematics that the mentors would be using)
2. Videotape Demonstration of a Complete Initial Interview done by myself which was meticulously "torn-apart" and analyzed (mapping the entire interview out on a large whiteboard with facilic symbols)
3. Videotape Demonstration Continued
4. Understanding the Power of Our Words (an introduction to the DOC supervision system that the mentors would be using to help the residents achieve an objective understanding of their frequency of open-ended questions, frequency of leading questions, and style of empathic engagement)

Day 2:

1. The Creative Use of Object Relations in the Initial Interview: The Importance of Psychodynamics
2. Interviewing Techniques for Uncovering Personality Dysfunction on Axis II of the DSM-IV (with video demonstration)
3. Uncovering Sensitive and Taboo Material: An Introduction to Five Interviewing Techniques for Improving Validity (with video demonstration)

4. Uncovering Suicidal Ideation and Intent: The Chronological Assessment of Suicide Events—the CASE Approach (with video demonstration)

At the end of the year-long mentorship, there was a third all-day workshop that was hosted at the residency director's house and was handled more as a retreat. In its final format it included three workshops: (1) "Transforming Confrontational Resistance: Angry Exchanges and Awkward Personal Questions from Patients," (2) An interactive group session focusing on an understanding of the personal impact and meaning of suicide on families, staff, and oneself (we pushed the residents to uncover their personal biases about suicide and how these biases could impact on their interviewing styles and their ability to spot suicidal patients), and (3) "How to Talk with Patients About Their Spirituality." We made a point of familiarizing residents with a variety of appropriate responses for handling difficult questions such as, "Dr. Shea, do you believe in God?" We felt that unless residents felt comfortable handling this question, they would be hesitant to ask patients about their religious beliefs. At the end of the retreat, we spent an hour garnering feedback from the residents on how we could improve the year-long mentorship.

The mentorship began with the mentor and resident meeting for an hour to discuss what the mentorship would be like and agreeing on a set time to meet for 2 hours every other week. Then the resident would make a videotape of an initial 50-minute intake. The mentor would review the intake by himself or herself and carefully map the interview out using facilics, noting such things as the use of empathy and engagement skills, the degree of open-endedness, the resident's nonverbals, and the resident's approach to specific clinical tasks such as eliciting suicidal ideation and performing a differential diagnosis using the *DSM-IV*.

At this point, the mentor and resident would meet for 2 hours to go over the videotape and develop an individualized learning program with two to four specific, mutually agreed-upon interviewing techniques, as areas for focused attention. Learning goals were operationalized and described by specific terms such as decreasing the number of "phantom gates," increasing the number of "natural gates," and utilizing "gentle assumption," etc.

The specificity of the supervision terms was greatly appreciated by residents. They reported that the well-defined supervision language made it easy for them to see what specifically needed to be done. Moreover, once they did it they could subsequently see their progress, providing a positive feedback loop which further motivated them to work harder on their interviewing. After goals were set in the initial meeting, it was agreed that the mentor would subsequently help the trainee master these skills. As the year progressed, once mastery was accomplished, new goals were set. Both in the initial videotape review and in ongoing mentorship, we emphasized positive re-enforcement.

From this point onwards, the mentor and trainee began to meet during the agreed-upon 2-hour blocks every other week. In the first hour of the sessions, the mentor would observe the resident doing a full initial intake interview in the clinic with the mentor in the room.

As the interview proceeded, the mentor would map out the interview with facilics and note everything from psychodynamics and structuring techniques to the resident's nonverbals and style of questioning using the DOC language, always carefully attending to the agreed-upon areas for improvement. By being in the room, the mentor could have the opportunity to demonstrate a specific interviewing strategy for the resident with the actual patient, providing a powerful learning experience. In the second hour, the mentor would provide feedback and coaching on what had just occurred. Role-playing was used to help consolidate specific interviewing techniques.

The resident was urged to continue to focus upon their agreed-upon interviewing goals in all subsequent interviews between mentoring sessions (a 2-week span). Some residents did this informally; others actually kept a "behavioral self-monitoring form" of their progress in the interviews performed between mentoring sessions. The self-monitoring form was then reviewed by the mentor at the beginning of each 2-hour block.

This self-monitoring approach helped residents understand that much of the work of the training program—practicing techniques—actually would occur outside the mentoring sessions, during their clinical interviews between sessions. It would be during these between-session interviews that much of the most productive work and improvement would occur, a process that parallels a psychotherapy patient's learning that much of the real work of therapy occurs between sessions (a point not missed by residents interested in doing psychotherapy).

Unlike the WPIC program, the very first interview was done by the mentor so that the resident would see a second clinician (my videotape presented in the First Day workshop being the first clinician) perform an initial interview from front to back, including observing nitty-gritty details such as how the mentor takes notes and why. As mentioned earlier, the willingness of the mentor to put herself or himself "on the spot" frequently helped break the ice in the mentorship dyad, especially if the mentor made some mistakes and openly discussed how she or he could have done the interview differently.

Throughout the year-long coaching, the mentor would refer the resident back to readings from the textbook that seemed particularly germane to the patient just interviewed or could help clarify or consolidate a technique that seemed confusing. For instance, if the patient exhibited subtle signs of psychosis that the resident did not recognize, then the resident would be referred to the chapter on interviewing techniques for uncovering psychotic process. In the next session of role-playing (as described below), the mentor and trainee could discuss aspects of the chapter and then role-play appropriate techniques.

If a patient did not show up as scheduled (happened about one third of the time), the 2 hours would be devoted to role-playing the specific techniques the resident had chosen to develop or that patient interactions had brought to light as areas of interest.

It was also during one of these "no-shows" that the mentor could conveniently role-play a patient with suicidal ideation and ask the resident to demonstrate the effective use of the CASE Approach to ensure that residents were competent in eliciting suicidal ideation (in future weeks, as the mentor observed the resident interviewing actual patients, the mentor could note whether the resident had successfully incorporated the CASE Approach into their ongoing work). Over the course of the year, most residents were observed doing about 10 to 15 actual interviews, with the other sessions being filled with role-playing.

The biggest disadvantage of the DIMP program was the loss of an ongoing multidisciplinary class, where trainees observed each other interviewing and shared feedback. Fortunately, the textbook emphasized multidisciplinary techniques, but the actual class interaction was a definite loss when compared to the WPIC program.

In our opinion, this loss was far outweighed by the significantly more comprehensive nature of the mentoring process, which received high praise from the residents. The longitudinal mentoring and diversity of patient presentations, the development of specific goals for improvement, the ability to practice and consolidate these goals by role-playing, and the richness of the relationship that developed over the year between mentor and resident were invaluable. To boot, providing mentorship was great fun, with most mentors finding the vivid interactive quality and the ability to actually see the resident's skills improve in front of them, highly enjoyable.

In addition to concrete improvements in interviewing skills, many of the residents seemed to gain a variety of intangibles such as increased confidence, increased excitement about interviewing, and, in many cases, an improvement in his or her ability to have an observing ego while interviewing (an ability that proved to be a boon to their development as psychotherapists as well).

In the 15 years of running the program, only a handful of residents balked at the process. In these cases, issues such as insecurity, social anxiety, or passive-aggressive tendencies seemed to make direct supervision more threatening. Fortunately, the longitudinal quality of the mentorship sometimes allowed the mentor to help the resident overcome these obstacles, while in a few instances, important deficiencies in the resident's skill or attitude were uncovered and brought to the attention of the residency director for intervention.

POTENTIAL MISTAKES IN COURSE DESIGN AND HOW TO AVOID THEM
Required Course Versus Optional

From our experience we have become convinced that you should always make sure that the clinical interviewing course and mentorship is required. At both WPIC and Dartmouth, an optional format was tried briefly. In both instances, the results were dismal. If the course is made optional, it can metacommunicate that interviewing is not *that* important. It is obvious to residents that the residency course in psychopharmacology is not optional, and if the interviewing course is optional, the resident has to wonder about the importance of the topic.

Moreover, even the most motivated of residents can be appropriately hesitant about being directly observed, and they are also frequently dealing with heavy workloads. Consequently, even some of the better trainees may not sign up or may slowly drop out because "I'm just so busy right now." Finally, the residents who may most need the training—residents with weak interviewing skills—will probably be the least likely to sign up for the course.

PGY-I versus PGY-II versus PGY-III

From our set of core principles, you will recall the importance we placed on scheduling the program at a time when residents are doing outpatient assessments (one of the single most critical factors for success of the program). The first year that we implemented the course at Dartmouth, we placed it in the PGY-II, thinking "the sooner the better" with regards to providing residents training in interviewing. At Dartmouth, these residents were primarily on inpatient units, and we found that they just "didn't quite get" the tight time constraints of a "50-minute hour" nor the specific difficulties unique to outpatient settings. Moreover, they were still so early in their training that they were somewhat flooded with information to learn and also lacked much of the observing ego that is useful for maximizing direct supervision. We then took this exact same group of residents and gave them interviewing mentors in PGY-III. Almost all of them said this time frame provided a significantly better learning experience.

If your outpatient experience is primarily in PGY-II, then the mentoring program is best suited there. It simply depends on the scheduling of this type of clinical experience in your residency program.

On the other hand, we now lean towards placing some components of interviewing training at differing time points in the residency. For instance, very shortly after completing their medical internship, as they begin their actual psychiatric training, we think it is a great time to give the residents the didactics (including video demonstrations if available) on validity techniques and the elicitation of suicidal ideation by methods such as the CASE Approach, as they are beginning their "on-call" duties.

First, this early exposure to key interviewing skills may significantly improve their ability to deliver quality emergency room care or quality interventions on inpatient units late at night while being "on-call." Second, it provides the resident, firsthand, with personal experience that interviewing techniques can be immensely practical and useful in their everyday work, thus priming them to be interested in interviewing as the residency continues. This may also be a good time to give the residents whatever textbook you choose on psychiatric interviewing, so that interested residents can read and obtain a theoretical framework for their early interviewing practice.

In PGY-II, if you have the capabilities to have a series of didactic classes as in the WPIC program, this can provide valuable information while stoking interest in learning about interviewing. Chapters from the book can be given as required reading, week by week, and discussed in the course. Such a structured setting greatly increases the likelihood that the trainees will both do and enjoy the reading as well as learn from each other.

If an appropriate outpatient experience also is available during PGY-II, then you could simultaneously run the year-long mentorship program. If not, the PGY-II classroom course would be followed by the mentoring program in PGY-III. Such a set-up might almost be ideal, providing residents with an extended interviewing focus that moved with the resident throughout the first three years of training.

PGY-IV residents, who were particularly excited about interviewing, can be trained as interviewing mentors and attend the interviewing mentor's monthly meetings. This was done at Dartmouth and the residents found it to be a powerful experience, some of whom later became full-time faculty and official mentors. Once again there is no right way, but these are suggestions to get you started.

One Mentor Versus Multiple Mentors

At the WPIC program there was only one teacher and mentor—me! This greatly limits the number of hours of mentoring each resident receives. It also jeopardizes the longevity of the program if your mentor leaves. Keep in mind, you can still provide an excellent experience with just one person, as was done at WPIC, and you may not have a choice because of limited faculty availability.

On the other hand, if at all possible, try to utilize multiple mentors, which can greatly increase the amount of direct supervision. If you do this, remember the importance of providing for the ongoing recruitment and training of new mentors, for suddenly a group of mentors may disappear, leaving the program precariously short-staffed, a problem we encountered at Dartmouth. We now realize that ongoing recruitment must be built into the program. Having PGY-IV residents (often chief residents) become mentors is one way of approaching this problem, for some residents stay to become faculty, often subsequently volunteering to become interviewing mentors.

Also remember the importance of the monthly mentor meetings. Although requiring time, we view these meetings as critical for maintaining the viability of the program over time. Mentorship is time consuming and can be frustrating in those rare occasions when you have a problematic resident. The camaraderie, cohesiveness, and joint problem- solving of supervision problems provided by the monthly mentor meetings is valuable in attracting and keeping mentors. All mentors must be required to attend.

SUMMARY

Always keep in mind the value of flexibility. Each residency brings with it, its own limitations in resources and its own potentials for creative solutions to those limitations. In any given residency one must determine which educational techniques may be most cost effective. Depending on the availability of resources, the core principles outlined in this article can be implemented in varying fashions. For instance, one program might meet the need for a well-grounded theoretical foundation through the use of didactics, a textbook, and supplemental readings. Another program might meet this need without the use of lectures, using a small-group seminar format and a textbook instead.

In the long run, one of the major goals of any interviewing training program is to stimulate intellectual excitement about the interviewing process. It is hoped that this excitement will involve residents in an ongoing exploration of their interviewing styles, that will continue until the very last interview of their careers. Only if this openness for future learning has been achieved can a clinical interviewing program fulfill its promise. As Sir William Osler [31] astutely observed, "The hardest conviction to get into the mind of a beginner is that the education upon which he is engaged is not a college course, not a medical course, but a life course, for which the work of a few years is but a preparation."

APPENDIX A

EDUCATIONAL GOALS LIST FOR PSYCHIATRIC INTERVIEWING SKILLS

In the following educational goals list (EGL), we have tried to present a state-of-the-art and comprehensive listing of the key concepts and techniques related to interviewing skills that we feel can be of immediate use to a resident in everyday clinical practice. The list is garnered from various readings and has been derived across various mental health disciplines.

We hope that it provides an unusually rich, "one-stop-shop" for both mentors and residents to become aware of all the exciting developments that are occurring in clinical interviewing. The list can be used throughout the mentorship to help the resident become aware of areas of interest that can be tapped as personalized interviewing goals, while suggesting resources for achieving those very same goals. As the year proceeds, the mentor and resident can review the list to check on progress. We also find that mentors sometimes discover—as we did—ideas and strategies on the EGL that are also new to them and prove to be useful areas for further exploration.

We also feel that you will find that some of the skill sets are particularly amenable to role-playing for acquisition and consolidation. For example, under "G: Handling Confrontational Resistance and Intense Affect," role-playing may be the single best modality for training the resident. Other interviewing skills that are particularly amenable to role-playing include: handling awkward questions or demands, handling challenges to clinician competence, working with hostile comments, recognizing and calming the potentially violent patient, working with tearful patients, reassuring the anxious or frightened patient, and working with patients exhibiting guarded or paranoid affect.

It is not expected that every resident, at the time of graduation from the residency, will be competent in using all of the interviewing skills listed under each goal category, but we do feel that by the time of graduation a resident should be competent in all of the lettered goals, choosing whichever specific techniques they and their mentors find necessary to achieve this competence. The EGL provides a resource where residents can become familiar with the many techniques designed to accomplish these goals, be aware of their personal strengths regarding their use, and spot areas for ongoing improvement within these core skill groups. In short, the EGL provides the resident with a convenient listing of key interviewing skills for ongoing growth both during the residency and throughout his or her career.

A. Psychodynamic interviewing skills
   1. Recognition of defense mechanisms
   2. Techniques of unstructured interviewing
   3. Elicitation of psychogenetic history and dynamic diagnosis
   4. Recognition of the seeds of transference and countertransference
   5. Assessment for psychotherapy
   6. Ability to recognize and use one's own feelings, associations, and fantasies
   7. Development of the clinician's observing ego
   8. Use of object relations and the psychology of the self in the initial interview
   9. Familiarization with key authors such as Sigmund Freud, Harry Stack Sullivan, John Whitehorn, Roger MacKinnon, Robert Michels, Leston Havens, Otto Kernberg, Heinz Kohut, Aaron Lazare, and others
B. Basic engagement skills
   1. Use of empathic statements
   2. Use of stroking and supportive statements
   3. Nonverbal facilitatory techniques (such as head nodding and eye contact)
   4. Study of proxemics (use of space)
   5. Study of kinesics (use of gesturing and body movement)
   6. Paralanguage skills (tone of voice and other speech characteristics)
   7. Recognition of weak or pathologic engagement
   8. Note taking
   9. Familiarization with key authors such as Edward Hall, Gerard Egan, Alfred Benjamin, Carl Rogers, Rita and John Sommers-Flanagan, and others
C. Advanced engagement skills
   1. Familiarity with leading theorists in collaborative interviewing such as Borden and Prochaska (four stages of change: 1. Precontemplation, 2. Contemplation, 3. Preparation, and 4. Action)
   2. Solution-focused interviewing
   3. Motivational interviewing (Miller and Rollnick)
   4. Medication interest model (Shea): how to talk with patients about their medications in a fashion designed to improve medication adherence
   5. Counterprojection and soundings (Leston Havens)
D. Understanding response modes: how clinicians phrase questions and statements
   1. Familiarity with major theorists in response mode clinical research such as Clara Hill
   2. Familiarity with the degree of openness continuum (DOC) Shea: open-ended questions, gentle commands, swing questions, qualitative questions, statements of inquiry (leading questions), empathic statements, facilitatory statements, closed-ended questions, and closed-ended statements

E. Basic and advanced structuring techniques
  1. Facilic supervision and schematics (Shea)
  2. Creating a conversational style while gathering large databases
  3. Understanding regions (content and process regions)
  4. Understanding transitions called "gates" (spontaneous gates, natural gates, referred gates, implied gates, phantom gates, and introduced gates)
  5. Attending to the changing needs of the patient depending on the structural phase of the interview (eg, introduction, opening, body of the interview, closing, and termination)
  6. Flexible strategies for structuring the interview depending upon time constraints and clinical tasks
F. Handling stylistic resistance
  1. Focusing loquacious and/or wandering patients
  2. Opening up reticent or shut-down patients
  3. Derailing rehearsed or manipulative interviews
  4. Effectively engaging patients with a formal thought disorder or mania
G. Handling confrontational resistance and intense affect
  1. Handling awkward questions or demands
  2. Handling challenges to clinician competence
  3. Working with hostile comments
  4. Recognizing and calming the potentially violent patient
  5. Working with tearful patients
  6. Reassuring the anxious or frightened patient
  7. Working with guarded or paranoid affect
H. Minimizing bias created by the interviewer
  1. Avoiding phrasing bias as seen with negative questions, cannon questions, leading questions, or overly wordy questions
  2. Avoiding nonverbal bias
I. Maximizing validity while probing sensitive areas
  1. Use of behavioral incidents (Gerald Pascal)
  2. Use of other validity techniques such as: gentle assumption (Pomeroy et al), induction to bragging (Othmer and Othmer), shame attenuation (Shea), normalization (Shea), symptom amplification (Shea), and denial of the specific (Shea)
  3. Familiarization with the uncovering techniques of neurolinguistic programming (Grinder and Bandler)
J. Phenomenologic inquiry (Jaspers) and descriptive psychopathology
  1. Basic techniques of phenomenological interviewing
  2. Understanding the patient's core psychologic pains
  3. Understanding the phenomenology of common forms of psychopathology such as organic syndromes, psychosis, mania, depression, obsessions and compulsions, posttraumatic stress disorder, substance abuse, eating disorders, and characterological problems
K. Exploring religion, spirituality, worldview, and framework for meaning
  1. Importance of exploring spirituality
  2. The potential impact of the interviewer's worldview on the interview
  3. The propriety of sharing one's own worldview with the patient: the advantages and disadvantages of self-disclosure
  4. Indirect methods of raising worldview
  5. Direct methods of raising worldview

   6. Interviewing techniques for an in-depth exploration of worldview
   7. Gracefully handling the patient's question, "Do you believe in God?"
   8. Familiarity with leading theorists such as Allan Josephson, John Peteet, and the Griffiths
L. Diagnostic skills
   1. Familiarity with multiaxial approaches in general and particularly the *DSM-IV-TR*
   2. Familiarity with *DSM-IV-TR* diagnostic criteria
   3. Ability to elicit symptoms relevant to specific *DSM-IV-TR* diagnoses on both Axis I and Axis II thoroughly but naturally
   4. Ability to recognize diagnostic leads
   5. Ability to use time constraints effectively and flexibly while exploring diagnostic criteria sensitively
   6. Ability to elicit an organized and accurate chronology of the history of the present illness
   7. Ability to uncover characterological disorders
   8. Ability to uncover family psychopathology
   9. Familiarity with key diagnostic interviewing theorists: Danny Carlat, Othmer and Othmer, David Robinson, James Morrison, and Shawn Christopher Shea
M. Content exploration
   1. Delineating the chief complaint, referral source, the history of the present illness, past psychiatric history, social history (including occupational, educational, relationship and childhood abuse histories), family history, general medical history, and review of physical systems
N. Suicide assessment
   1. Eliciting risk and protective factors
   2. Understanding and using the Chronological Assessment of Suicide Events (CASE) Approach (Shea, 1998)
      a. Presenting suicide events (last 48 hours)
      b. Recent suicide events (last 2 months)
      c. Past suicide events
      d. Immediate suicide events (now/next)
O. Assessment of sensitive and taboo material
   1. Rape and assault
   2. Spouse, parent, and child abuse
   3. Antisocial behavior
   4. Normal and pathologic sexual/gambling history
   5. Drug and alcohol history
   6. Treatment and medication nonadherence
P. Interviewing techniques related to cultural diversity issues
   1. Nonverbal considerations related to culture and the interview
   2. Differences in greeting related to culture
   3. Varying taboos about sharing psychiatric concerns related to culture and questions used to sensitively explore such issues
   4. Differing approaches to discussing treatments and medications related to culture
Q. Talking with family members of patients who have severe mental illnesses
   1. Interviewing techniques for decreasing stigma
   2. Interviewing techniques for decreasing shame and guilt
   3. Interviewing techniques for decreasing biases and fears about mental health professionals

4. Interviewing techniques for helping family members understand and respond appropriately to patient symptoms such as obsessions and compulsions, non-lethal self injury such as self-cutting, and suicidal behavior
5. Interviewing techniques for helping family members deal with the death of a loved one by suicide
6. Interviewing techniques for psychoeducation about mental illnesses and treatment interventions from medications to psychotherapy

R. Interviewing techniques related to the mental status
1. Familiarization with key descriptive terms such as loosening of associations, tangential speech, circumstantial speech, restricted affect, inappropriate affect, flat affect, the difference between mood and affect, among others
2. Techniques used for cognitive testing including the Folstein Mini-Mental Status
3. Techniques for helping patients to feel less shame and guilt related to deficits uncovered during cognitive testing
4. Familiarization with key theorists such as Strub and Black, David Robinson, Trezpacz and Baker

APPENDIX B

CORE COURSE OUTLINE FOR PSYCHIATRIC INTERVIEWING

The following course syllabus is an example, in our opinion, of a comprehensive and powerful introduction to the art of clinical interviewing. If you have the resources it can be used as a direct model for your own curriculum.

Naturally, resources are limited, and they can even change, within a single institute over time, as faculty come and go. Consequently, we also designed this curriculum to provide a practical platform for helping course designers to create shorter courses in an organized and informed fashion. This list can help the designer to pick and choose classes, having a better idea of the pros and cons (eg, what exactly will be lost) by the deletion of certain topics. A review of the list may also suggest how some classes, for the sake of time limitations, might be combined. For example, the two separate classes on cultural diversity and exploring spirituality might be combined comfortably into a single class.

We feel that, when guided by an organized decision-making process, a director can create a sound introductory course on clinical interviewing in as few as 10 classes. If you are faced with such a tough decision, we hope this model curriculum can help you to creatively design a course syllabus that nicely fits the needs and limitations of a particular institute. (By the way, anytime you can use videotape or DVD demonstrations of your techniques, the class is invariably improved).

Section 1: Cornerstone Principles of Clinical Interviewing

Class 1: Introduction: the primary importance of engagement
Key topics include:

    Goals of clinical interviewing
    Engagement

Blending; unconditional positive regard (Carl Rogers)
Sullivan's "engagement question" and his concept of the "self-system"
Collaborative interviewing strategies including solution-focused interviewing
Motivational interviewing (Miller and Rollnick)

Class 2: The language of interviewing
Key topics include:

Facilic supervision (a language for understanding how to structure the interview
sensitively)–(Shea)
The Degree of Openness Continuum (DOC)—a language for understanding
nine different types of clinician responses (open questions, statements of gentle command, swing questions, qualitative questions, facilitatory statements,
statements of inquiry, empathic statements, closed questions, and closed
statements)–(Shea)

Class 3: The structure of the interview: traps, roadblocks, strategies and solutions
Key topics include:

Five phases of the interview
Scouting phase
Clinician analysis during opening minutes of the interview
Issues during the introduction and closing phase
Transforming initial resistance
Sensitively structuring the interview
Creating a conversational mode
Cross-sectional facilic diagrams (strategies for managing the four quadrants of
time used for gathering information)
Recognizing problematic interview such as the shut-down interview and the
wandering interview

*Class 4: Videotape/DVD demonstration of an initial interview: part I (requires about
1.5 hours)*
This class is a videotaped demonstration of an entire initial interview, done by
one of the mentors, which the class analyzes and discusses by collaboratively
mapping out the interview on a large whiteboard using facilic schematics. All
aspects of the interview are discussed, including:

Engagement techniques
Psychodynamic issues
Differential diagnosis by the *DSM-IV-TR*
Gathering of all major content regions from social history to the medical history
Mental status
Lethality assessment
Nonverbal communication

*Class 5: Videotape/DVD demonstration of an initial interview: part II (requires
about 1.5 hours)*
This class is a continuation of Class 4, focusing on the second half of the demonstration interview

Class 6: Transforming the shut-down interview
Key topics include:

> Differing reasons the shut-down process emerges, ranging from anxiety to oppo-
> sitional behavior
> Use of the principles of the DOC to transform shut-down interviews
> Specific methods for engaging reticent patients
> Role-playing exercises

Class 7: Sensitively structuring the wandering patient
Key topics include:

> Differing reasons for wandering to emerge, ranging from histrionic process to
> hypomania
> Use of the understanding of the DOC and closed-ended techniques to focus the
> patient
> Appropriate use of cut-offs
> Avoiding "the dead zone" for data gathering
> Effective use of time as related to clinical tasks
> Role-playing exercises

Class 8: Nonverbal behavior
Key topic include:

> Proxemics (Edward Hall)
> Kinesics (Ray Birdwhistell)
> Paralanguage and tone of voice
> Facial expression
> Eye contact
> Clues to deceit
> Seating arrangement
> Note taking
> Displacement activities
> Postural echoing

Section 2: Psychopathology and the Interview Process

Class 9: Exploring depression and mania
Key topics include:

> Phenomenology of mood disturbance
> Critical data for *DSM-IV-TR* diagnosis
> Techniques for eliciting data about mood symptoms including depression, ma-
> nia, and mixed states
> Questions for uncovering hypomania as seen in bipolar types II, III, and IV

Class 10: Exploring anxiety symptoms
Key topics include:

> Phenomenology of anxiety symptoms
> Critical data for *DSM-IV-TR* diagnosis

Techniques for eliciting data about anxiety symptoms, picking up atypical panic attacks and atypical flashbacks in posttraumatic stress disorder, sensitive questions for screening for obsessive-compulsive disorder

Class 11: Exploring substance abuse and eating disorder symptoms
Key topics include:

Phenomenology of substance abuse
Approaches to minimization and denial
The CAGE: a four-question quick screen for alcohol abuse
Interviewing techniques for delineating a *DSM-IV-TR* diagnosis
Phenomenology of eating disorders
Techniques for delineating a *DSM-IV-TR* diagnosis of an eating disorder

Class 12: Exploring psychotic process
Key topics include:

Phenomenology of psychotic process
The life cycle of a psychosis
Schneiderian first rank symptoms and questions for spotting them
Critical data for *DSM-IV-TR* diagnosis
Soft signs of psychosis
Engagement techniques for eliciting data pertinent to psychotic symptoms

Class 13: Exploring personality dysfunction
Key topics include:

The role of the social history in the diagnosis of Axis II disorders
Deflecting defensive resistance typical of some people who have Axis II disorders in the initial interview
Typical defense mechanisms
Signal signs
Signal symptoms
Probe questions
The two-step strategy for delineating diagnoses on Axis II of the *DSM-IV-TR*

Class 14: The cognitive mental examination as related to delirium and dementia
Key topics include:

Orientation techniques
Digit spans
Vigilance test
Trails test
Four-object recall
Constructions
The Folstein Mini-Mental Status
Humanistic concerns during the cognitive examination

Section 3: Advanced Interviewing Techniques and Psychodynamic Interviewing Perspectives:

Class 15: Vantage points: bridges to psychotherapy
Key topics include:

Attentional vantage point
Use of fantasy and clinician countertransference
Harry Stack Sullivan and participant observation
The observing ego and self-remembering
Conceptual vantage points

Class 16: Validity techniques: interview techniques for uncovering sensitive and taboo topics
This class describes interviewing techniques for uncovering the truth about domestic violence, incest, antisocial behavior, substance abuse, suicide and homicide, and medication nonadherence including:

The behavioral incident
Normalization
Shame attenuation
Induction to bragging
Gentle assumption
Symptom amplification
Denial of the specific
The uncovering techniques of Grinder and Bandler

Class 17: Interviewing techniques for sensitively eliciting suicidal behaviors, ideation, and intent
Key topics include:

Phenomenology of suicide
Uncovering risk and protective factors
Interviewing techniques for probing "dangerous material"
Chronological Assessment of Suicide Events (CASE) approach—an interview strategy for eliciting suicidal ideation, intent, and behaviors (Shea)
Triad of lethality
Documentation of suicide assessments

Class 18: Role-playing workshop on transforming resistance and gracefully handling awkward patient questions
Key topics include:

Strategically sliding on the oppositional continuum
Natural methods of transforming anger
"Pulling resistance"
Strategic empathy
Avoiding the "paranoid spiral"
Leston Haven's counterprojection

Side-tracking
Content responses
Process responses

Class 19: Assessment for dynamic psychotherapy
Key topics include:

Desirable patient characteristics
Understanding the "process" of patient behavior and the patient's response to interpretive questions
Use of reflecting statements
Questions that help one choose the time-limited psychotherapy best suited to the unique characteristics of the patient

Class 20: Introduction to the role of the psychodynamic formulation
Key topics include:

Psychogenetic history
Spotting defense mechanisms
Identifying unconscious conflict
Identification
Projective identification
Introjection
Incorporation
Kernberg's structural interviewing

Class 21: The use of object relations and the psychology of the self in the initial interview
Key topics include:

Normal and abnormal development of the self
Part-self/part-object
Merger object
Self-objects
Split affects
Otto Kernberg
Heinz Kohut
The bipolar self
The effective use of complementary shifts

Section 4: Special Topics Requiring Specific Interviewing Skills

Class 22: Interviewing techniques related to cultural diversity
Key topics include:

Nonverbal considerations
Differences in greeting related to culture
Varying taboos about sharing psychiatric symptoms and how to navigate them
Differing approaches to discussing treatments and medications related to culture

Class 23: Exploring religion, spirituality, worldview, and framework for meaning
Key topics include:

Familiarity with leading theorists such as Allan Josephson, John Peteet, and the Griffiths
Importance of exploring spirituality
Potential impact of the interviewer's worldview on the interview
Advantages and disadvantages of self-disclosure
Indirect methods of raising worldview
Direct methods of raising worldview
Gracefully handling the patient's question, "Do you believe in God?"

Chapter 24: Improving medication adherence: how to talk with patients about their medications
Key topics include:

Why patients don't take medications
The medication interest model (Shea)
The choice triad
Interviewing techniques based on the medication interest model such as
    The inquiry into lost dreams
    The inquiry into medication sensitivity
    The trap-door question
Dismantling the crutch myth
The question of efficacy
The question of cost
The question of what taking medications symbolizes to the patient

Chapter 25: Talking with family members of patients having severe mental illnesses
Key topics include:

Interviewing techniques for reducing stigma
Interviewing techniques for decreasing shame and guilt
Interviewing techniques for decreasing biases and fears about mental health professionals
Interviewing techniques for helping families understand and respond appropriately to patient symptoms such as obsessions and compulsions, nonlethal self-injury such as self-cutting, and suicidal behaviors
Helping family members deal with the death of a loved one by suicide
Familiarity with leading theorists including Aaron Murray-Swank, Lisa Dixon, Bette Stewart, Robert Drake, and Kim Mueser

References

[1] Sullivan HS. The psychiatric interview. New York: W.W. Norton company; 1970.
[2] Langsley DC, Hollender MH. The definition of a psychiatrist. Am J Psychiatry 1982;139: 81–5.
[3] Langsley DC, Yager J. The definition of a psychiatrist: eight years later. Am J Psychiatry 1988;145:469–75.
[4] Shea SC, Mezzich JE, Bohon S, et al. A comprehensive and individualized psychiatric interviewing training program. Acad Psychiatry 1989;13(2):61–72.

[5] Engler CM, Saltzman CA, Walker ML, et al. Medical student acquisition and retention of communication and interviewing skills. J Med Educ 1981;56:572–9.
[6] Levinson W, Roter D. The effects of two continuing medical education programs on communication skills of practicing primary care physicians. J Gen Intern Med 1993;8: 318–24.
[7] Shea C. Contemporary clinical interviewing: integration of the DSM-IV, managed care concerns, mental status, and research. In: Goldstein G, Hersen M, editors. Handbook of psychological assessment. 3rd edition. New York: Pergamon; 2000.
[8] Shea SC. Psychiatric interviewing. In: Sledge WH, Warren C, editors. Core readings in psychiatry. Washington, DC: American Psychiatric Press, Inc.; 1995.
[9] Shea SC, Mezzich JE. Contemporary psychiatric interviewing: new directions for training. Psychiatry, Interpersonal and Biological Processes 1988;51(4):385–97.
[10] Carlat DJ. The psychiatric interview: a practical guide. 2nd edition. New York: Lippincott Williams & Wilkins; 2004.
[11] MacKinnon RA, Michels RM, Buckley PJ. The psychiatric interview in clinical practice. 2nd edition. Washington, DC: American Psychiatric Publishing, Inc.; 2006.
[12] James M. The first interview: revised for DSM-IV. New York: Guilford; 1995.
[13] Othmer E, Othmer SC. The clinical interview using DSM-IV TR. Vol 1: fundamentals Washington, DC: American Psychiatric Publishing, Inc.; 2002.
[14] Shea SC. Psychiatric interviewing: the art of understanding. 2nd edition. Philadelphia: W.B. Saunders Company; 1998.
[15] Sommers-Flanagan R, Sommers-Flanagan J. Clinical interviewing. 3rd edition. New York: John Wiley & Sons, Inc.; 2002.
[16] Pascal GR. The practical art of diagnostic interviewing. Homewood (IL): Dow Jones-Irwin; 1983.
[17] Miller W, Rollnick S. Motivational interviewing: preparing people to change addictive behavior. New York: Guilford Press; 1991.
[18] Shea SC. The delicate art of eliciting suicidal ideation. Psychiatr Ann 2004;34:385–400.
[19] Shea SC. The chronological assessment of suicide events: a practical interviewing strategy for eliciting suicidal ideation. J Clin Psychiatry 1998;59(Suppl 20):58–72.
[20] Shea SC. The practical art of suicide assessment: a guide for mental health professionals and substance abuse counselors. New York: John Wiley & Sons, Inc.; 2002.
[21] Shea SC. The chronological assessment of suicide events (the CASE approach): an introduction for the front-line clinician. NewsLink [the Newsletter of the American Association of Suicidology]. Fall 2003;29,2.
[22] Available at: EndingSuicide.com. [a centralized suicide prevention education site funded by the National Institute of Mental Health, contract #N44MH22045] provides details on the use of the CASE Approach.
[23] Magellan behavioral health care guidelines. CASE approach recommended to participating clinicians. 2002.
[24] Shea SC. Practical tips for eliciting suicidal ideation for the substance abuse professional. Counselor, the Magazine for Addiction Professionals 2001;2(6):14–24.
[25] Shea SC. Tips for uncovering suicidal ideation in the primary care setting. In: Hidden diagnosis: uncovering anxiety and depressive disorders (version 2.0) [four-part CD-Rom series]. GlaxoSmithKline; 1999.
[26] Innovations in the elicitation of suicidal ideation: the chronological assessment of suicide events (CASE approach). Presentation for the Federal Bureau of Prison's Annual Meeting of Chief Psychologists. Tucson (AZ), 2001.
[27] Innovations in the elicitation of suicidal ideation: the chronological assessment of suicide events (CASE approach). Presentation for the Federal Bureau of Prison's Annual Meeting of Psychiatrists. Atlanta (GA), 2003.
[28] Shea SC. Improving medication adherence: how to talk with patients about their medications. Philadelphia: Lippincott Williams & Wilkins; 2006.

314 SHEA, GREEN, BARNEY, ET AL

[29] Josephson A, Peteet J, editors. Handbook of spirituality and worldview in clinical practice. Washington, DC: American Psychiatric Publishing, Inc.; 2004.
[30] Griffith JL, Griffith ME. Encountering the sacred in psychotherapy: how to talk with people about their spiritual lives. New York: Guilford; 2002.
[31] Osler W. Aequanimitas. 3rd edition. Philadelphia: Blakiston; 1945.

INDEX

A

Alcohol history, eliciting, 220–221

Alliance with families, in inpatient settings, disruptive issues for clinicians in, 170–172
    confidentiality concerns, 171–172
    time limitations, 171
    emotional responses to illness and hospitalization in, 168–169
    expectations of treatment in, 169–170
    fears, anxieties, and concerns of, 168–170
    roles and determination of spokespersons in, 170
   in outpatient settings, 172–179
    differences in opinion on helping patient, 173–174
    fears, anxieties, concerns of, 172–175
    problems establishing rapport and reliable contact with treatment team in, 174–175
    unmet needs for information in, 172–173
   obstacles for clinician, engaging family members in treatment, 178–179
    talking with patients about family involvement in care, 176–178
   of patients with mental illness, **167–180**

Antisocial behavior, behavioral incident technique and, 253–254
   uncovering, **253–259**

Anxiety, about oral board patient examinaion, 203–204
   about role-play, e42–e45
   distractibility and poor concentration in, 236–237
   of families with mentally ill member, 168–170, 172–175

Attention-deficit hyperactivity disorder, distractibility *vs.,* 236–237

B

Behavioral incident technique, anchor questions in, e14
   fact finding style of, 253
   illustrative dialogue for, 257–258
   in antisocial behavior and suicide assessments, 253–254
   in chronological assessment of suicide events, e12
   in creation of verbal videotape, e13–e14
   role-play of, e17
   sequencing style in, e12–e14, 254
   uses of, e22–e23

Beliefs, of difficult patient, 245–246
   of interviewer, 183–184
   worldview as, 192–193, 292

Biopsychosociospiritual model, in matrix treatment planning, 183

Bipolar disorder, diagnostic quandries in, tips for, **233–238**
   mania in, symptom differentiation in, 234–237

Boundaries, clinician self-disclosure and, 185
   psychologic safety and, 152

C

Chronological Assessment of Suicide Events (CASE Approach), 259, 290–291

Chronological Assessment of Suicide Events (CASE Approach), behavioral incident in, e12–e14
   denial of the specific in, e14–e15
   description of, e12–e14, e16
   development of, e10
   gentle assumption in, e14–e15
   in literature, e10
   interviewing techniques in, e11–e12
   macrotraining of, e16–e20
    benefits of, e19–e20
    maps of regions, e16
    performance of Regions 1 and 2 in, e19
    preparation for, e16
    Region 1 in, e17
    Region 2 in, e14–e15, e17–e18
    Region 3 in, e19
    Region 4 in, e19

Note: Page numbers of article titles are in **boldface** type.

0193-953X/07/$ – see front matter
doi:10.1016/S0193-953X(07)00043-3

Moving?

Make sure your subscription moves with you!

To notify us of your new address, find your **Clinics Account Number** (located on your mailing label above your name), and contact customer service at:

E-mail: elspcs@elsevier.com

800-654-2452 (subscribers in the U.S. & Canada)
407-345-4000 (subscribers outside of the U.S. & Canada)

Fax number: 407-363-9661

Elsevier Periodicals Customer Service
6277 Sea Harbor Drive
Orlando, FL 32887-4800

*To ensure uninterrupted delivery of your subscription, please notify us at least 4 weeks in advance of move.

ELSEVIER